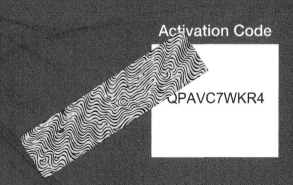

BROWN'S REGIONAL ANESTHESIA REVIEW

BROWN'S REGIONAL ANESTHESIA REVIEW

Ehab Farag, MD, FRCA

Associate Professor and Director of
Clinical Research
Cleveland Clinic Learner College of
Medicine
Staff Anesthesiologist
Anesthesiology Institute
Cleveland Clinic
Cleveland, OH

Loran Mounir-Soliman, MD

Director, Acute Pain Service
Director, Regional Anesthesia
Fellowship
Staff Anesthesiologist
Anesthesiology Institute
Cleveland Clinic
Cleveland, OH

ILLUSTRATIONS BY
Joe Kanasz

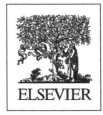

ELSEVIER

ELSEVIER

1600 John F. Kennedy Blvd.
Ste 1800
Philadelphia, PA 19103-2899

BROWN'S REGIONAL ANESTHESIA REVIEW   ISBN 978-0-323-40056 5

Notice

Knowledge and best practice in this field are constantly changing. As new research and experience broaden
our knowledge, changes in practice, treatment, and drug therapy may become necessary or appropriate.
Readers are advised to check the most current information provided (i) on procedures featured or (ii) by the
manufacturer of each product to be administered, to verify the recommended dose or formula, the method
and duration of administration, and contraindications. It is the responsibility of the practitioner, relying on
his or her own experience and knowledge of the patient, to make diagnoses, to determine dosages and the best
treatment for each individual patient, and to take all appropriate safety precautions. To the fullest extent of
the law, neither the Publisher nor the Authors assume any liability for any injury and/or damage to persons or
property arising out of or related to any use of the material contained in this book.

Library of Congress Cataloging in Publication Data
A catalog record for this book is available from the Library of Congress.

Executive Content Strategist: Bill Schmitt
Content Development Specialist: Carole McMurray
Project Manager: Julie Taylor
Illustrations Manager: Karen Giacomucci
Designer: Christian Bilbow

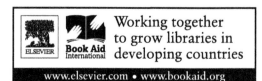

To my daughter, Monica, who has been an inspiration and joy in my life.

Ehab Farag

I dedicate this book to an amazing woman, my wife Dalia, whose relentless support is my real strength. To Natalie, Krista, and Nicole, the true joys of my life, and last but not least, my mom whose prayers bless my steps.

Loran Mounir-Soliman

Contents

Preface

Regional anesthesia has become a distinctive specialty in anesthetic practice. However, despite its importance for anesthetic practice, there is no dedicated review book for regional anesthesia. Therefore, we designed this review book to be a companion to *Brown's Atlas of Regional Anesthesia*. This review is unique, for applied anatomy, ultrasound techniques, complications, and pitfalls pertinent to every block have been covered in addition to the pharmacology of local anesthetics in adults and pediatric patients. Furthermore, for the first time, there is a chapter dedicated solely to the neurological complications of regional anesthesia based on the latest ASRA report on neurological complications associated with regional anesthesia. This review will be an invaluable tool for reviewing the subject of regional anesthesia for anesthesiology residents, regional anesthesia fellows, and practicing anesthesiologists. If readers are interested in more information, they can refer to *Brown's Atlas of Regional Anesthesia*.

We would like to express our gratitude to our colleagues who helped write this review and to the editorial assistants Ms. Mariela Madrilejos from the Cleveland Clinic and Ms. Carole McMurray from Elsevier.

Ehab Farag, MD, FRCA
Loran Mounir-Soliman, MD
Cleveland, Ohio, 2015

Contributors

Maria Bauer, MD
The University of Texas Health
Science Center at Houston,
MvGovern Medical School
Houston, TX

Devin S. Caswell, DO MD
Department of Anesthesiology
Cleveland Clinic Foundation
Cleveland, Ohio

Kenneth C. Cummings III, MD MS
Medical Director, PACE Clinic and OnePACC
Department of General Anesthesiology
Cleveland Clinic
Cleveland, Ohio

Suzanne Dupler, DO
Department of Anesthesiology
Cleveland Clinic Foundation
Cleveland, Ohio

Hesham Elsharkawy, MD, MSc
Assistant Professor of Anesthesiology
General Anesthesiology, Pain Management, Outcomes
    Research, Anesthesiology Institute
CCLCM, Case Western Reserve University
Cleveland, Ohio

Ibrahim Farid, MD
Associate Professor of Anesthesiology, NEOMED
Chair, Department of Anesthesia and Pain Medicine
Director, Pediatric Pain Center
Akron Children's Hospital
Akron, Ohio

John George, III, MD
Assistant Professor of Anesthesiology
Cleveland Clinic
Cleveland, Ohio

Hari Kalagara, MD
Department of Anesthesiology
Cleveland Clinic Foundation
Cleveland, Ohio

Rami Karroum, MD
Assistant Professor of Anesthesiology, NEOMED
Department of Anesthesia and Pain Medicine
Akron Children's Hospital
Akron, Ohio

Sree Kolli, MD
Department of Anesthesiology
Cleveland Clinic Foundation
Cleveland, Ohio

Kamal Maheshwari, MD MPH
Staff Anesthesiologist
Acute Pain Management
Cleveland Clinic Foundation
Cleveland, Ohio

Hashim J. Qureshi, DO
Anesthesiology Institute
Cleveland Clinic Foundation
Cleveland, Ohio

Wael Ali Sakr Esa, MD PhD
Assistant Professor of Anesthesiology
General Anesthesiology, Pain Management
Director Orthopedic Anesthesia
Anesthesiology Institute
CCLCM, Case Western Reserve University
Cleveland, Ohio

John Seif, MD
Department of Pediatric Anesthesiology
Cleveland Clinic
Cleveland, Ohio

Mark Teen, MD
Department of Anesthesiology
Cleveland Clinic Foundation
Cleveland, Ohio

Maria Yared, MD
Assistant Professor of Anesthesiology
Department of Anesthesia and Perioperative Medicine
Medical University of South Carolina
Charleston, South Carolina

CHAPTER 1

Pharmacology

Kamal Maheshwari

Questions
Local anesthetics

1. Which of the following local anesthetics is metabolized by a pseudocholinesterase?

   A. Lidocaine
   B. Mepivacaine
   c. Procaine
   D. Prilocaine

2. According to the manufacturer of Depobupivacaine (Exparel), which of the following statements regarding drug administration is incorrect?

   A. The maximum dosage should not exceed 266 mg (one 20 mL vial).
   B. Exparel can be mixed with other local anesthetics prior to injection.
   c. Vials of Exparel should be inverted to resuspend the particles immediately prior to withdrawal from the vial.
   D. Exparel should be used within 4 hours of preparation in a syringe.

3. An early sign of local anesthetic toxicity is:

   A. Lightheadedness and dizziness
   B. Muscle twitching and convulsions
   c. Cardiovascular depression and collapse
   D. Respiratory depression and arrest
   E. Hypotension

4. According to the American Society of Regional Anesthesia and Pain Medicine, treatment of local anesthetic toxicity includes:

   A. Epinephrine doses less than 1 mcg/kg
   B. Lipid emulsion (20%) bolus 1.5 mL/kg (lean body mass) intravenously, followed by continuous infusion 0.25 mL/kg/min
   c. Repeat bolus once or twice for persistent cardiovascular collapse
   D. Decrease the infusion rate to 0.1 mL/kg/min if blood pressure remains low.
   E. All of the above

5. Which of the following statements is true about local anesthetic cardiac toxicity?

   A Bupivacaine is the most cardiotoxic drug.
   B. Lipid solubility and high protein binding of bupivacaine are factors responsible for higher cardiotoxicity.
   c. The R(+) isomer very avidly binds to cardiac sodium channels.
   D. Bupivacaine does not release from a binding site easily.
   E. All of the above

6. The true statement for using dexamethasone as an additive to local anesthetic is:

    A. Dexamethasone prolongs the duration of analgesia but not the motor blockade.
    B. Dexamethasone prolongs the duration of analgesia and the motor blockade.
    C. Perineural dexamethasone decreases the incidence of postoperative nausea and vomiting (PONV).
    D. Dexamethasone addition helps in only intermediate-acting local anesthetics.

7. Local anesthetic has the greatest affinity for:

    A. Beta subunit of voltage-gated sodium channels in the open state
    B. Beta subunit of voltage-gated sodium channels in the resting state
    C. Alpha subunit of voltage-gated sodium channels in the inactivated state
    D. Beta subunit of voltage-gated sodium channels in the inactivated state
    E. Alpha subunit of voltage-gated sodium channels in the resting state

8. The true statement reflecting mechanism of action of local anesthetic is:

    A. Local anesthetic blocks the alpha subunit of sodium channels on the extracellular surface.
    B. Ionized form of local anesthetic crosses the lipid membrane easily.
    C. Local anesthetic binds to the sodium channel more avidly in the nonionized state.
    D. Sodium channels in the activated or inactivated have greater affinity for local anesthetics than in the resting state.
    E. All of the above

9. Which of the following is true regarding systemic absorption of local anesthetics?

    A. Addition of epinephrine reduces systemic absorption and increases toxic dose.
    B. Systemic absorption is not dependent on the dose of local anesthetic.
    C. Intercostal is greater than tracheal.
    D. Paracervical is greater than caudal.
    E. Sciatic is greater than brachial.

10. The true statement about methemoglobinemia is:

    A. It is a reduction of hemoglobin to methemoglobin.
    B. It is associated with administration of prilocaine and benzocaine but not with Cetacaine and lidocaine.
    C. Methemoglobin cannot bind oxygen or carbon dioxide, resulting in loss of the hemoglobin molecule's transport function.
    D. Methemoglobin normally constitutes 5% of the total hemoglobin.

11. Which of the following statements is true regarding local anesthetic physical properties?

    A. Local anesthetics are weak acids.
    B. The pKa of local anesthetics is between 5.5 and 7.5.
    C. Local anesthetics are highly soluble as unprotonated amines.
    D. Local anesthetics are generally marketed as hydrochloride salts that are slightly acidic.

12. The true statement regarding metabolism of local anesthetics is:

    A. Ester local anesthetics are metabolized by plasma esterases.
    B. Amide local anesthetics are metabolized by liver, primarily hydrolysis by cytochrome enzymes.
    C. Termination of action of local anesthetic in spinal cord (spinal anesthesia) is by systemic absorption.
    D. Reduced cardiac output will not affect metabolism of amide local anesthetic.
    E. Both A and C
    F. All of the above

13. Which of the following statements is true?

    A. Lidocaine is an amide local anesthetic.
    B. Eutectic mixture of local anesthetics (EMLA) has lidocaine (2.5%) and prilocaine (2.5%).
    C. Lidocaine is metabolized in the liver to monoethylglycine and xylidide.
    D. Monoethylglycine and xylidide have local anesthetic properties.
    E. All of the above

14. The true statement about intravenous regional anesthesia (Bier's block) is:

    A. Lidocaine (0.5%) is the drug of choice (max: 4 mg/kg).
    B. Early tourniquet deflation can lead to systemic toxicity.
    C. The action of local anesthetics on both nerve ending and nerve trunks is presumptive mechanism of action.
    D. Prilocaine can be used and has a lower margin of safety.
    E. Choices A, B, and C
    F. All of the above

15. Which of the following statements is true regarding use of lidocaine in the perioperative period?

    A. Lidocaine has antiinflammatory properties.
    B. The antiinflammatory effect of lidocaine is due to the reduction in inflammatory mediators signaling (e.g., inhibition of platelet activating factor).
    C. Lidocaine inhibits neutrophil accumulation at the site of inflammation and impairs free radical release.
    D. Lidocaine has bacteriostatic properties.
    E. All of the above

Answers

1. **(C)** Amide local anesthetics are lidocaine, mepivacaine, and prilocaine, and they all are metabolized by P450 enzymes in the liver. Ester, like procaine, is metabolized by pseudocholinesterases.

2. **(B)** Exparel should not be mixed with any other local anesthetic, although it can be diluted with normal saline.

3. **(A)** Manifestations of local anesthetic toxicity typically appear 1 to 5 minutes after the injection. Classically, systemic toxicity begins with symptoms of CNS excitement, such as circumoral and/or tongue numbness, metallic taste, lightheadedness, dizziness, visual and auditory disturbances (difficulty focusing and tinnitus), disorientation, and drowsiness. With higher doses, initial CNS excitation is often followed by a rapid CNS depression, with the following features: muscle twitching, convulsions, unconsciousness, coma, respiratory depression and arrest, cardiovascular depression, and collapse.

4. **(A, B, and C)** Answers A, B, and C are part of the checklist for Treatment of Local Anesthetic Systemic Toxicity. Option D is incorrect. The recommendation is to double the infusion rate to 0.5 mL/kg/min if the blood pressure remains low.

5. **(E)** All the statements are true.

6. **(B)** Addition of dexamethasone with local anesthetic solutions in peripheral nerve blocks prolongs the durations of analgesia and motor blockade. These effects were documented with both intermediate and long-acting local anesthetics. In addition, perineural administration of dexamethasone decreased the incidence of PONV. (Reference PMID—25774458).

7. **(C)** Local anesthetics bind avidly to voltage-gated sodium channels in active and inactivated state. They have low affinity for sodium channels in the resting phase.

8. **(D)** Local anesthetic blocks alpha subunit of sodium channel by attaching to the intracellular surface. The nonionized form (lipid soluble) crosses the lipid membrane, and once intracellular, local anesthetic molecule converts into the ionized form (water soluble). It is the ionized form that attaches to the channel intracellular surface. Neurons that are active have sodium channels in an active or inactive state, compared with a resting state. Local anesthetic binds avidly to sodium channel in active neuron, not the resting neurons.

9. **(A)** The addition of epinephrine causes local vasoconstriction and reduces systemic absorption. This leads to more drugs being available at the site, increasing the toxic dose as more drugs can be given. A higher dose leads to higher systemic absorption. Absorption of local anesthetics depends on the type of the block: tracheal > intercostal > caudal > paracervical > epidural > brachial plexus > sciatic.

10. (C) It is the oxidation of hemoglobin that results in the formation of methemoglobin. The local anesthetics prilocaine, benzocaine, Cetacaine, and lidocaine all can induce methemoglobinemia. Methemoglobin cannot bind oxygen or carbon dioxide, resulting in loss of the hemoglobin molecule's transport function. Methemoglobin normally constitutes less than 1% of the total hemoglobin.

11. (D) Local anesthetics are weak bases, with pKa ranging from 8 to 9. The pKa is the pH of the solution at which local anesthetics are equally divided in protonated and unprotonated form. Local anesthetics are weak bases that are mostly unprotonated and not very soluble. They are stored and marketed as slightly acidic solutions (hydrochloride salts) because it makes them water soluble, and acidic solution helps stabilize additives like epinephrine. Once injected in the tissues the pH of local anesthetic solution rapidly equilibrates with that of the surrounding area.

12. (E) Ester local anesthetics are metabolized by plasma esterases. Amide local anesthetics are metabolized by cytochromes in the liver first in dealkylation and then hydrolysis. There are no esterases in the spinal cord and the termination of action of local anesthetic is due to systemic uptake. Reduced cardiac output will reduce hepatic blood flow and can reduce metabolism of amide local anesthetics.

13. (E)

14. (E) Intravenous regional anesthesia is a commonly used technique for short upper extremity procedures. The limb is exsanguinated with the help of a tourniquet and local anesthetic is injected in the vein. Amide (lidocaine, mepivacaine, ropivacaine, prilocaine) can be used, but lidocaine is a commonly used drug. The local anesthetic acts on nerve ending and nerve trunks to produce anesthesia. Prilocaine has lower plasma concentration compared to lidocaine after tourniquet deflation, signifying lower systemic toxicity and higher margin of safety.

15. (E) Local anesthetics have antiinflammatory properties that are not mediated through sodium channel blockade but through inhibition of inflammatory cytokine signaling. Also, local anesthetic inhibits neutrophil accumulation and activation. Local anesthetics also have bacteriostatic properties.

CHAPTER 2

Pharmacology of Pediatric

Rami Karroum and Ibrahim Farid

Questions

1. Amide local anesthetics (LAs) are metabolized in the liver by cytochrome P450 enzymes. These enzymes reach adult activity level by:

    A. 9 to 12 months
    B. 20 to 24 months
    C. 36 months
    D. 48 months

2. Amide LAs bind to serum proteins, α_1-acid glycoprotein and albumin. Infants have a decreased level of α_1-acid glycoprotein and albumin. Adult levels of protein binding are reached at about:

    A. 6 months
    B. 9 months
    C. 12 months
    D. 18 months

3. Neonates and infants are more sensitive than adults to amide LAs induced cardiotoxicity due to their:

    A. Relatively larger volume of distribution (VD) of amide LAs compared to adults
    B. Higher baseline heart rates
    C. Lower clearance
    D. Lower protein binding

4. EMLA cream (eutectic mixture of local anesthetics) application in excess of the maximum recommended allowable dose, particularly in neonates, can result in:

    A. Hemolytic anemia
    B. Jaundice
    C. Methemoglobinemia
    D. Hypoxia

5. Neonates require larger doses of LAs for spinal anesthesia, and the duration of the spinal block is shorter compared with adults due to:

    A. Larger total volume of CSF
    B. More rapid turnover of CSF than in adults
    C. A and B
    D. Higher glucose content of CSF

6. Levobupivacaine carries a reduced risk of cardiac toxicity compared with bupivacaine due to:

    A. It contains a higher amount of D-enantiomer than bupivacaine.
    B. It contains a higher amount of L-enantiomer than bupivacaine.
    C. It contains only L-enantiomer.
    D. It contains only D-enantiomer.

7. Chloroprocaine is increasingly used to provide continuous epidural infusion for postoperative pain control in neonates instead of amide LAs because:

    A. It is rapidly metabolized by cholinesterases.
    B. It is rapidly metabolized by the liver.
    C. It is rapidly eliminated by the kidney.
    D. It has higher binding to albumin.

8. In pediatric patients, the earliest and most sensitive sign of unintentional intravascular injection of LAs, when mixed with epinephrine (usually in 1/200,000 dilution), is:

    A. Increase in systolic blood pressure more than 10%
    B. Increase T wave amplitude more than 50% compared to baseline and ST segment changes
    C. Increase in heart rate 10 to 15 beats above baseline heart rate
    D. Seizure

9. Which of the following nerve block is associated with the highest absorption of local anesthetics?

    A. Supraclavicular nerve block
    B. Femoral nerve block
    C. Intercostal nerve block
    D. Sciatic nerve block

10. The maximum recommended dose of ropivacaine in toddlers is:

    A. 2 mg/kg
    B. 3 mg/kg
    C. 4 mg/kg
    D. 5 mg/kg

11. The maximum rate of infusion of epidural bupivacaine in neonates should not exceed:

    A. 0.1 mg/kg/hr for no more than 48 hours
    B. 0.2 mg/kg/hr for no more than 48 hours
    C. 0.3 mg/kg/hr for no more than 48 hours
    D. 0.4 mg/kg/hr for no more than 48 hours

12. When two different LAs are mixed together, their individual toxicity and maximal allowable dose are:

    A. Additive
    B. Potentiated
    C. Reduced
    D. Not changed

13. The recommended initial bolus of intralipid 20% for treatment of LAs induced cardiotoxicity in pediatric patients is:

    A. 0.25 mL/kg
    B. 0.5 mL/kg
    C. 1.5 mg/kg
    D. 2.5 mg/kg

14. In pediatric patients, amide LAs induced systemic toxicity presenting signs compared to adults is:

    A. Similar
    B. Cardiac toxicity precedes CNS toxicity.
    C. CNS toxicity precedes cardiac toxicity.
    D. Both CNS and cardiac toxicity occur simultaneously.

15. The maximum dose of 2-chloroprocaine is:

    A. 5 mg/kg
    B. 10 mg/kg
    C. 15 mg/kg
    D. 20 mg/kg

Answers

1. (A) Amide local anesthetics (LAs) are metabolized in the liver by cytochrome P450 enzymes. These enzymes reach adult activity level by 9 to 12 months. Therefore, neonates and infants have a higher serum-free fraction of amide LAs and are more prone to develop toxicity.

2. (C) Adult levels of protein binding are reached at about 12 months. Therefore, neonates and infants are more prone to develop toxicity from amide LAs due to a higher serum-free fraction.

3. (B) Direct cardiac toxicity is due to prolonged blockade of the sodium channels in the cardiac conduction system, resulting in a profound decrease in ventricular conduction velocity. The susceptibility to cardiac toxicity is amplified by increased heart rates. Neonates and infants are more sensitive than adults to amide LAs induced cardiotoxicity due to their higher baseline heart rates.

4. (C) EMLA cream is a eutectic mixture of equal quantities of lidocaine 2.5% and prilocaine 2.5%. It is commonly used to provide transdermal local anesthesia in pediatric patients. Methemoglobinemia has been reported with the use of EMLA cream. Therefore, the maximum total surface area to which the cream is applied should be calculated in advance, and the maximum allowable dose should never be exceeded. This is particularly important in neonates.

5. (C) Neonates have a larger total volume of CSF compared to adults (4 mL/kg compared to 2 mL/kg, respectively). In addition, 50% of the total CSF volume is in the spinal portion of the subarachnoid space compared to only 25% of the total CSF volume in adults. Also, neonates have a more rapid turnover of CSF than do adults. As a result, neonates require larger doses of LAs for spinal anesthesia, and the duration of the spinal block is shorter.

6. (C) Levobupivacaine has almost the same blocking properties and pharmacokinetics as its racemic counterpart bupivacaine. The effect on the cardiac conduction system is stereo-specific, with the L-enantiomer having much less effect than the D-enantiomer present in the racemic mixture of bupivacaine. As a result, levobupivacaine carries a reduced risk of cardiac toxicity compared to bupivacaine.

7. (A) Chloroprocaine is increasingly used to provide continuous epidural infusion for postoperative pain control in neonates. It is rapidly metabolized by cholinesterases, with an elimination half-life of a few minutes. Although neonates have a reduced level of plasma esterases compared to adults, this is clinically insignificant. Therefore, the incidence of systemic toxicity is rare and the risk of accumulation is minimal. This safety profile allows better analgesia in neonates as it allows the use of higher infusion rates and thus wider dermatomal coverage compared with amide LAs.

8. (B) Order of sensitivity for detection of unintentional intravascular injection in pediatric, from most to least sensitive: increase in T wave amplitude and ST segment changes > increase in systolic blood pressure greater than 10% > increase in heart rate 10 to 15 beats. After the age of 8 years, T wave changes are less sensitive for detection of intravascular injection.

9. (C) Absorption of LAs from the site of regional block from higher to lower: intercostal > caudal > lumbar epidural > thoracic epidural > brachial > femoral > sciatic.

10. (B)

11. (B)

12. (A) When mixing two different LAs, toxicity is additive. So, when mixing equivalent amounts of two different local anesthetics, the maximum dose for each should be reduced by 50%.

13. (C) Pediatric dose is similar to adult doses and consists of a bolus of 1.5 mL/kg over 1 minute. Repeat bolus dose can be given in 3 to 5 minutes with a maximum of 3 mL/kg. This is followed by a maintenance infusion of 0.25 mL/kg/min until the circulation is restored.

14. (B) In pediatrics, signs of cardiac toxicity may precede signs of CNS toxicity or may be the only sign of systemic toxicity. This is different from adults, in which signs of CNS toxicity usually precede cardiac toxicity.

15. (D)

Bibliography

Karroum, R.E., Farid, I., 2017. Pharmacology of Local Anesthetics In Pediatrics. In: Farag, E., Mounir-Sosliman, L. (Eds.), Brown's Atlas of Regional Anesthesia, fifth ed. Elsevier, Philadelphia, pp. 17–22.

CHAPTER 3

Interscalene Block

Hashim J. Qureshi

Questions

1. You are asked to perform an interscalene block for shoulder surgery on an otherwise healthy 55-year-old male. In order to successfully perform the block, which landmarks would you use to identify the posterior triangle?

   A. Posterior border of the sternocleidomastoid and trapezius muscles at the level C6 and C7 vertebrae
   B. Medial border of the sternocleidomastoid and trapezius muscles at the level of C5 and C6 vertebrae
   C. Medial border of the anterior scalene and anterior border of the sternocleidomastoid muscle at the level of C6 and C7 cervical vertebrae
   D. Posterior border of the sternocleidomastoid muscle at the level of C5 and C6 vertebrae
   E. None of the above

2. Why do the nerve roots of C5, C6, and C7 appear as hypoechogenic nodules under ultrasound when scanning between the anterior scalene and middle scalene underneath the prevertebral fascia?

   A. Equal ratio of neural to nonneural tissue
   B. Higher ratio of nonneural to neural tissue
   C. Higher ratio of neural to nonneural tissue
   D. Lower ratio of neural to nonneural tissue
   E. None of the above

3. You are utilizing ultrasound to perform an interscalene block on an elderly female who is about to undergo a right total shoulder arthroplasty. How would you identify the dorsal scapular and the long thoracic nerves while scanning for the brachial plexus under ultrasound at the proper level?

   A. 2 cm anterior to the brachial plexus located in the anterior scalene
   B. 1 cm anterior to the brachial plexus located in the middle scalene
   C. 2 cm posterior to the brachial plexus located in the anterior scalene
   D. Less than 1 cm posterior to the brachial plexus located in the middle scalene
   E. Less than 1 cm anterior to the brachial plexus located in the anterior scalene

4. You are asked to evaluate a 40-year-old male in the postanesthesia care unit who had a left interscalene catheter placed for a shoulder revision and is now having pain along his clavicle and his anteromedial shoulder that is not being covered by the nerve block. What nerve is not being covered by the interscalene catheter?

   A. Suprascapular nerve
   B. Dorsal scapular nerve
   C. Musculocutaneous nerve
   D. Supraclavicular nerve
   E. Axillary nerve

5. After surgery to repair a right humeral fracture, a 43-year-old female patient with an interscalene nerve block is complaining of pain along her medial forearm and hand. What nerve could have possibly been missed with the nerve block?

   A. Radial nerve
   B. Ulnar nerve
   C. Intercostobrachial nerve
   D. Median nerve
   E. Musculocutaneous nerve

6. What is the best way to reduce phrenic nerve involvement while performing an interscalene block?

   A. Puncture localization 1 to 2 cm cranial to the cricoid cartilage
   B. Puncture localization 1 to 2 cm caudal to the cricoid cartilage
   C. Puncture localization at the level of the C7 vertebra
   D. Puncture localization 2 to 3 cm cranial to the C7 vertebra
   E. None of the above

7. A few days after needle insertion into the middle scalene muscle for an interscalene block, your patient presents with a right side ache along the medial border of the scapula and a physical exam is remarkable for the right scapulae being farther from midline when compared to the left. What nerve has most likely been injured?

   A. Dorsal scapular
   B. Long thoracic
   C. Supraclavicular
   D. Intercostal
   E. Axillary nerve

8. What could an injury to the long thoracic nerve while performing an interscalene block present as?

   A. Chronic pain of the shoulder and weakness of the serratus posterior muscle
   B. Chronic back pain and weakness of the trapezius muscle
   C. Chronic pain of the shoulder and weakness of the serratus anterior muscle
   D. Chronic back pain and weakness of the serratus anterior muscle
   E. None of the above

9. A 38-year-old male has received an interscalene block for a left shoulder arthroplasty resulting in a dense block along his arm, hand, and the majority of his shoulder except the upper portion. What can be done to add to the block?

   A. Injecting local anesthetic around C3 to C4 nerve roots
   B. Injecting local anesthetic around C8 to T1 nerve roots
   C. Performing an intercostobrachial block
   D. Repeating the interscalene block
   E. None of the above

10. Where should the nerve catheter be positioned in order to have a high chance of a successful surgical shoulder block?

   A. C7 to C8 nerve roots
   B. C5 to C6 nerve roots
   C. C4 to C5 nerve roots
   D. C8 to T1 nerve roots
   E. None of the above

11. What patient population is most susceptible to adverse events from an interscalene nerve block?

    A. 58-year-old male smoker with severe chronic obstructive pulmonary disease (COPD)
    B. 21-year-old female with exercise-induced asthma
    C. 75-year-old male with mild coronary artery disease
    D. 25-year-old female in her first trimester of pregnancy
    E. 37-year-old male with sickle cell trait

12. The most common complication associated with an interscalene nerve block is:

    A. Vertebral artery injection
    B. Recurrent laryngeal nerve paralysis
    C. Phrenic nerve paralysis
    D. Internal carotid artery injection
    E. Pneumothorax

13. You are asked by the surgeon to perform an interscalene block for right hand surgery but you are hesitant to perform this procedure because:

    A. An interscalene block would be appropriate for this procedure.
    B. Upper cervical nerve roots would be spared.
    C. Lower cervical nerve roots would be spared.
    D. Upper and lower cervical nerve roots would both be spared.
    E. None of the above

Answers

1. (A) The interscalene block is most successfully performed utilizing the posterior triangle, which lies between the posterior border of the sternocleidomastoid and trapezius muscles, at the level of the sixth and seventh cervical vertebrae.

2. (C) The nerve roots of C5, C6, and C7 appear as hypoechogenic nodules due to the higher ratio of neural to nonneural tissue located at this level of the brachial plexus.

3. (D) The dorsal scapular and long thoracic nerves appear as hyperechoic structures with a hypoechoic center found in the middle scalene less than 1 cm posterior to the brachial plexus.

4. (D) The supraclavicular nerve arises from the C3 to C4 nerve roots and supplies sensory innervation to the cape of the shoulder.

5. (B) The interscalene block is most utilized for shoulder and humeral fracture surgeries but is not sufficient for surgeries involving the hand because the lower nerve roots and trunk of the brachial plexus are missed.

6. (B) The phrenic nerve and brachial plexus are within 2 mm of each other at the level of the cricoid cartilage (C6) and separate 3 mm for every 1 cm caudal from the cricoid cartilage; thus, puncture localization 1 to 2 cm caudal to the cricoid cartilage can help reduce phrenic nerve involvement with this procedure.

7. (A) Injury to the dorsal scapular nerve is characterized by a dull ache along the medial border of the scapulae along with weakness or hypotrophy of the rhomboid and levator scapulae muscles.

8. (C) Injury to the long thoracic nerve typically presents as chronic pain of the shoulder and weakness of the serratus anterior muscle, manifesting as the classic "winged scapula" when a patient pushes an outstretched hand against a wall.

9. (A) Injecting local anesthetic around C3 to C4 nerve roots would give you a superficial cervical plexus block and help this patient since these nerve roots supply some sensation to the upper parts of the shoulder.

10. (B) Proper positioning of the nerve catheter between C5 to C6 or C6 to C7 below the dorsal scapular and long thoracic nerves provides better anchoring space for the catheter, affording the highest chance for a successful nerve block.

11. (A) Due to the almost 100% involvement of the ipsilateral phrenic nerve with an interscalene block, it is advisable to be cautious with patients with limited pulmonary function such as patients with COPD.

12. (C) The most common complication associated with an interscalene block is involvement of the ipsilateral phrenic nerve; thus, caution must be taken with patients who have limited pulmonary function.

13. (C) Lower cervical nerve roots supplying the ulnar nerve are usually spared with the interscalene block, thus providing poor coverage for the medial forearm and hand.

CHAPTER 4

Supraclavicular Block

Devin S. Caswell

Questions

1. A 74-year-old patient had a recent fall and fractured her right proximal humerus. She is scheduled for an open reduction internal fixation, and regional anesthesia was requested by the surgeon. A peripheral nerve block was chosen to anesthetize the brachial plexus using the supraclavicular approach. In relation to the supraclavicular artery, where will the trunks and divisions lie while using ultrasound?

   A. Anterior and lateral
   B. Superior and lateral
   C. Superior and medial
   D. Superior and posterior
   E. Anterior and medial

2. A 35-year-old male is scheduled for shoulder arthroscopy at an ambulatory surgery center to evaluate pain he has developed from years of playing baseball. Regional anesthesia is performed targeting the brachial plexus using the supraclavicular approach. After the block, the patient has lost sensation of his arm and forearm as well as decreased motor function of his arm and hand. During the procedure, the patient complains of posterior shoulder pain. Which nerve was most likely not anesthetized, causing the patient's pain with this block?

   A. Subscapular nerve
   B. Suprascapular nerve
   C. Infrascapular nerve
   D. Intercostobrachial nerve
   E. Axillary nerve

3. A brachial plexus block is performed using the supraclavicular approach for shoulder surgery. A catheter will be placed for postoperative analgesia. For the most optimal analgesia in this patient, the catheter should be placed:

   A. Anterior to the subclavian artery
   B. Posterior to the subclavian artery
   C. Superior to the subclavian artery
   D. As close as possible to the first rib
   E. Under the first rib

4. A patient is scheduled for open reduction internal fixation of his fourth and fifth metacarpals after a fracture sustained during a fight. A brachial plexus block is performed using the supraclavicular approach and 10 cc of 0.1% ropivacaine was injected superior to the supraclavicular artery. Which one of these nerves is most likely spared by the block?

   A. Axillary nerve
   B. Musculocutaneous nerve
   C. Radial nerve
   D. Ulnar nerve
   E. Median nerve

5. A patient is scheduled for stage one creation of a dialysis fistula of the upper extremity because of his underlying chronic kidney disease (CKD). While undergoing a brachial plexus block using the supraclavicular approach, the patient suddenly develops chest pain and begins coughing. What is the best action that should be taken?

   A. Continue with the block.
   B. Place a catheter at this location.
   C. Stop the block and proceed with surgery under general anesthesia.
   D. Obtain a chest radiograph.
   E. Remove the needle and hold pressure.

6. After receiving a brachial plexus block with the supraclavicular approach, the patient undergoes shoulder arthroscopy; although experiencing numbness and weakness in the lower arm and hand, the patient develops severe shoulder pain. Which nerve was most likely affected, causing this pain?

   A. Suprascapular nerve
   B. Subscapular nerve
   C. Radial nerve
   D. Intercostobrachial nerve
   E. Infrascapular nerve

7. What is the most common complication associated with a brachial plexus block using the supraclavicular approach?

   A. Intravascular injection into the subclavian artery
   B. Intravascular injection into the vertebral artery
   C. Pneumothorax
   D. Failed block
   E. Phrenic nerve paralysis

8. Which section of the brachial plexus is anesthetized when performing a supraclavicular block?

   A. Roots and trunks
   B. Trunks and division
   C. Division and cords
   D. Cords
   E. Branches

9. What is the best indication for a supraclavicular block?

   A. Shoulder surgery
   B. Surgery of fifth digit
   C. Upper limb and hand surgery
   D. Shoulder arthroscopy
   E. First rib excision

10. Which of these patient positions is the optimal position for performing a supraclavicular block?

    A. Prone with a pillow under the chest
    B. Supine with the patient's head turned toward the side of the block
    C. Semisitting with the head of the bed at 45 degrees
    D. Semisitting with the head of the bed at 30 degrees
    E. Lateral recumbent with the block side up

11. After successfully performing a preoperative supraclavicular block for creation of an arteriovenous (AV) fistula, the anterior chest wall is scanned using ultrasound. When trying to rule out pneumothorax, what ultrasound sign should be present?

    A. Sliding sign
    B. Scaling sign
    C. Rolling sign
    D. Intrapleural air sign
    E. Friction rub

12. Which portion of the upper extremity may not be completely anesthetized after performing a supraclavicular block?

    A. Lateral portion of the hand

    B. Elbow

    C. Medial portion of the hand

    D. Posterior medial portion of the forearm

    E. Anterior lateral portion of the arm

13. A 38-year-old male presents to the operating room for ulnar nerve anterior transposition due to cubital tunnel syndrome not relieved by medial management. The surgeon requests regional anesthesia prior to starting the case. A brachial plexus block using the supraclavicular approach was performed with 30 cc of 0.75% bupivacaine prior to being transported to the operating room. Which one of these signs and/or symptoms is the first to present in local anesthetic toxicity?

    A. Seizure

    B. Lightheadedness

    C. Visual disturbances

    D. Hemodynamic collapse

    E. Shivering

Answers

1. (D) When using ultrasound, in the supraclavicular approach for the brachial plexus, the trunks and the divisions appear as a compact group of nerves (bunch of grapes) lying superior and posterior to the artery.

2. (B) Although the block can be used for shoulder surgery, it can miss the suprascapular nerve, which supplies the sensory innervation to the glenohumeral joint. Therefore, the block could fail to provide appropriate analgesia after shoulder surgery.

3. (C) The catheter is usually inserted superior to the subclavian artery in the case of shoulder surgery or in the corner pocket between the artery and first rib in the case of hand surgery. The correct position of the catheter can be confirmed under ultrasound by injecting local anesthetic or 1 mL of air into the catheter and observing the distribution in relation to the plexus.

4. (D) For the hand surgery, the local anesthetic should be inserted in the corner pocket between the subclavian artery and the first rib to avoid missing the lower trunk and its divisions and, therefore, the ulnar nerve.

5. (D) If the patient developed chest pain and cough during the procedure, the patient might have developed pneumothorax. The procedure should be abandoned and a chest x-ray should be ordered to confirm the diagnosis.

6. (A) Injury to the suprascapular nerve following supraclavicular block is usually presented by severe shoulder pain followed by weakness in supraspinatus and infraspinatus muscles. To avoid this complication, try not to inject above the plexus to avoid exposing the nerve to toxic high concentration of local anesthetics. In addition, avoiding injection above the plexus might decrease the incidence of phrenic nerve palsy after the block.

7. (E) To avoid phrenic nerve paralysis, try not to inject above the plexus to avoid exposing the nerve to toxic high concentration of local anesthetics. In addition, avoiding injection above the plexus might decrease the incidence of phrenic nerve palsy after the block.

8. (B) The brachial plexus in the supraclavicular region is composed mainly of three trunks: superior, middle, and inferior. These trunks pass across the upper surface of the first rib, where they lie posterior and superior to the subclavian artery. The trunks then divide into anterior and posterior divisions behind the clavicle.

9. (C) The supraclavicular block is very efficient for upper limb and hand surgeries.

10. (C) The patient could be in a semisitting position (beach chair) by elevating the head of the bed 45 degrees or the supine position with the patient's head turned to the opposite side to be blocked. The first position is preferable in obese patients.

11. (A) Try to examine the anterior chest wall by ultrasound after every supraclavicular block to confirm the absence of pneumothorax by the visualizing intact pleura (sliding sign).

12. (C) The block can be used for shoulder, elbow, or hand surgery; however, it can miss the lower portion of the brachial plexus, thus sparing the ulnar nerve distribution of the medial side of the hand.

13. (B) Local anesthetic toxicity typically occurs due to inadvertent intravascular or intrathecal injection or an excessive dosage leading to elevated blood concentrations of the drug. Initial signs and/or symptoms of local anesthetic toxicity include lightheadedness, dizziness, and numbness of the tongue. Further central nervous system (CNS) excitation can occur, manifesting as visual or auditory disturbances, shivering or muscle twitching, and, ultimately, seizure (generalized tonic-clonic seizures). Even higher plasma drug levels will lead to cardiovascular collapse.

CHAPTER 5

Axillary Block

Wael Ali Sakr Esa

Questions

DIRECTIONS (Questions 1 to 4): Please match the structure below with the letter that corresponds to it in the ultrasound image.

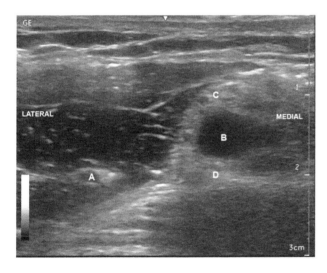

1. Musculocutaneous nerve _____

2. Axillary artery _____

3. Median nerve _____

4. Radial nerve _____

5. Axillary block can be used in all of these surgeries to control pain EXCEPT:

   A. Elbow surgeries
   B. Hand surgeries
   C. Wrist surgeries
   D. Shoulder surgeries
   E. Forearm surgeries

6. Inadequate anesthesia for the lateral part of the forearm following an axillary block is most likely the result of inadequate block to which nerve?

   A. Ulnar nerve
   B. Radial nerve
   C. Intercostobrachial nerve
   D. Median nerve
   E. Musculocutaneous nerve

7. Which nerve provides motor branches to the flexors of the hand and wrist?

   A. Median nerve
   B. Ulnar nerve
   C. Radial nerve
   D. Musculocutaneous nerve
   E. Intercostobrachial nerve

8. Complications of the axillary block include:

   A. Nerve injury
   B. Vascular puncture
   C. Hematoma
   D. Local anesthetic toxicity
   E. All of the above

9. All of the following statements are true about the radial nerve EXCEPT:

   A. It originates as a terminal branch of the medial cord.
   B. It leaves the axilla by passing below the teres major muscle.
   C. It supplies branches to the triceps, extensor radialis longus, and brachioradialis muscles.
   D. It innervates the lateral aspect of the arm.
   E. It innervates the posterior aspect of the forearm and hand.

10. Which nerve provides sensory innervation to the fourth and fifth digits?

    A. Median nerve
    B. Radial nerve
    C. Musculocutaneous nerve
    D. Intercostobrachial nerve
    E. Ulnar nerve

11. To avoid nerve injury while performing axillary block, which of the following should be taken into consideration?

    A. Avoid injection of local anesthetic when high resistance is encountered.
    B. Avoid injection of local anesthetic when simulation is obtained with intensity of less than 0.2 mA.
    C. Stop injecting the local anesthetic when the patient complains of severe pain during the injection of the local anesthetic.
    D. All of the above

12. Under ultrasound the musculocutaneous nerve appears as a:

    A. Hypoechoic circular nerve
    B. Hypoechoic flattened oval with a bright hyperechoic rim
    C. Hyperechoic flattened oval nerve with a hypoechoic rim
    D. None of the above

13. Under ultrasound, the relation of the median nerve to the axillary artery while performing the axillary brachial plexus block is:

    A. Superficial and medial to the artery
    B. Posterior and lateral to the artery
    C. Posterior and medial to the artery
    D. Superficial and lateral to the artery
    E. None of the above

14. All of the following statements are true about the axillary brachial plexus block relative to an interscalene brachial plexus block EXCEPT:

    A. It is relatively simple to perform under ultrasound.
    B. It lowers the risk of complications as compared with interscalene brachial plexus block.
    C. It can be used for surgical anesthesia for wrist surgeries.
    D. It can be used to control pain for shoulder surgeries.

15. All of the following statements are true about axillary brachial plexus block EXCEPT:

    A. Under ultrasound, the median nerve is a rounded hyperechoic structure.
    B. A curved ultrasound transducer probe should be used when performing the block.
    C. The structures of interest when performing the block are superficial, 1 to 3 cm from the skin.
    D. The axillary artery can be associated with one or more axillary veins and is usually located medially to the artery.

Answers

From 1 to 4, the structures on the ultrasound image are: **A**, **B**, **C**, **D**.

5. (D) An axillary block can provide excellent pain coverage for surgeries on the midarm down to the elbow, for elbow surgeries, and for wrist and hand surgeries. An axillary block will not provide pain control for shoulder surgeries. An interscalene block and a supraclavicular block provide excellent pain control for shoulder surgeries.

6. (E) The musculocutaneous nerve is a terminal branch of the lateral cord of the brachial plexus. Without blockade of the musculocutaneous nerve, adequate anesthesia of the lateral forearm is unlikely. Classic teaching is that the musculocutaneous nerve blockade can be accomplished by the injection of local anesthetic into the belly of the coracobrachialis muscle. Ultrasound studies have shown that the musculocutaneous nerve is not in the coracobrachialis muscle in approximately 20% of patients.

7. (A) The median nerve originates from both the medial and lateral cords. It provides motor branches to the flexors of the hand and wrist. It provides sensory innervation to the palmar surface of the first, second, and third digits and to the lateral half of the fourth digit.

8. (E) A hematoma can occur during an axillary block, especially if the patient was on an anticoagulant or if there are multiple needle punctures to the veins or axillary artery. The most common cause of local anesthetic systemic toxicity during axillary block is inadvertent intravascular injection. To avoid systemic toxicity during an axillary block, avoid fast forceful injection of local anesthetic, perform careful frequent aspiration during the injection, and adjust the dose and volume of local anesthetic injected in frail and elderly patients.

9. (A) The radial nerve is a terminal branch of the posterior cord. The radial nerve leaves the axilla by passing below the teres major and between the humerus and the long head of the triceps.

10. (E) The ulnar nerve is a terminal branch of the medial cord. The ulnar nerve has articular branches to the elbow joint and muscular branches to the hand and forearm. The ulnar nerve provides sensory innervation to the fourth and fifth digits.

11. (D) To avoid nerve injury during an axillary block, never inject local anesthetic when abnormal high resistance is encountered on injection, and stop injecting local anesthetic when patient complains of severe pain on injection and when simulation is obtained with current intensity of less than 0.2 mA. Withdraw the needle slightly to obtain the same response with current greater than 0.2 mA before injecting the local anesthetics.

12. (B) Under ultrasound, the musculocutaneous nerve has a characteristic appearance of a hypoechoic flattened oval with a bright hyperechoic rim.

13. (D) Surrounding the axillary artery are three of the four principal branches of the brachial plexus: the median nerve is superficial and lateral to the axillary artery; the ulnar nerve is superficial and medial to the axillary artery; and the radial nerve is posterior and lateral or posterior and medial to the axillary artery.

14. (D) The axillary brachial plexus block technique is relatively simple to perform using ultrasound. It is associated with a relatively lower risk of complications as compared with an interscalene block (as a vertebral artery puncture). Although individual nerves can be identified easily near to the axillary artery, it is not necessary as the deposition of the local anesthetic around the axillary artery is sufficient for an effective block.

15. (B) In order to obtain the best image when performing the axillary brachial plexus block, a linear transducer (8 to 14 MHz) should be used to obtain a higher resolution; a higher penetration is not needed as the structures of interest are superficial, 1 to 3 cm from the skin. A curved transducer should be used when imaging deeper structures as it allows higher penetration at the expense of lower resolution.

CHAPTER 6

Infraclavicular Block Review

Kenneth C. Cummings III

Questions

1. An infraclavicular block is typically performed at which level of the brachial plexus?

   A. Terminal nerves
   B. Cords
   C. Roots
   D. Divisions

2. Identify the starred structure in the ultrasound image. Cephalad is to the left.

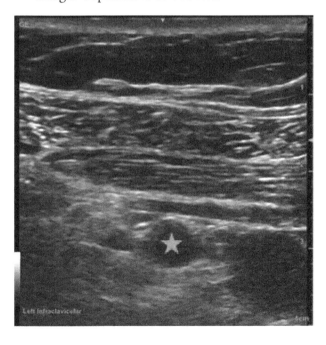

   A. Lateral cord
   B. Axillary vein
   C. Axillary artery
   D. Brachial artery

3. Identify the fascial plane indicated in the ultrasound image. Cephalad is to the left.

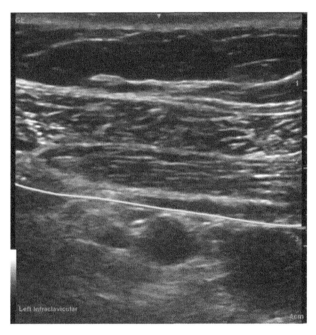

   A. Deltoid
   B. Pectoralis minor
   C. Endothoracic
   D. Fascia lata

4. A patient receives an infraclavicular block for radial fracture fixation. Complete anesthesia of the hand and forearm is noted. Upon inflation of the surgical tourniquet, the patient complains of pain under the axilla. Which nerve was not blocked?

   A. Musculocutaneous
   B. Radial
   C. Medial brachial cutaneous
   D. Intercostobrachial

5. Identify the numbered structures in order (1 to 3) in the image. Cephalad is to the left.

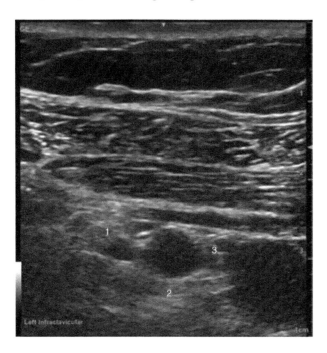

   A. Medial cord, lateral cord, posterior cord
   B. Median nerve, radial nerve, ulnar nerve
   C. Lateral cord, medial cord, posterior cord
   D. Lateral cord, posterior cord, medial cord

6. A patient has an infraclavicular catheter placed for analgesia after elbow arthroplasty. She received an initial bolus followed by continuous infusion. Approximately 12 hours after the block, she complains of severe pain on the lateral side of her elbow. Motor function in her hand is diminished. All tubing is connected and the pump is working. What is the most likely cause?

   A. Radial nerve injury from the block
   B. Normal postoperative pain
   C. Secondary block failure
   D. Incorrect drug choice

7. Advantages of infraclavicular blocks over axillary blocks include all of the following EXCEPT:

   A. Single needle entry
   B. Block of medial brachial cutaneous and medial antebrachial cutaneous nerves
   C. Easier catheter placement for continuous analgesia
   D. Ease of needle visualization with ultrasound

8. While determining the location for needle insertion for an infraclavicular block, the anesthesiologist is unable to visualize the axillary vessels or brachial plexus just medial to the coracoid process. The best course of action is:

   A. Abduct the arm and flex the elbow.
   B. Scan medially until the plexus is visible.
   C. Abandon the procedure because it is not possible in this patient.
   D. Use a nerve stimulator because the structures are too deep to image using ultrasound in this patient.

9. In the image, cephalad is to the left of the image. Between which two cords is local anesthetic being injected?

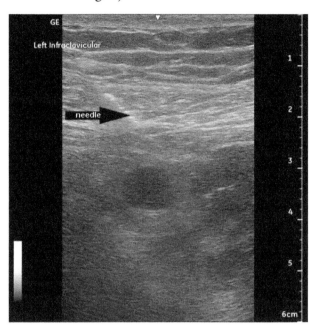

A. Medial and lateral
B. Posterior and lateral
C. Posterior and medial
D. Unable to determine

10. Methods to improve needle visualization during infraclavicular block include all of the following EXCEPT:

A. Observe tissue movement when moving the needle.
B. Use an echogenic (textured) needle.
C. Inject local anesthetic intermittently to improve visualization of the needle tip.
D. Angle the transducer or alter the applied pressure.

11. In the image, cephalad is left. A sample pattern of a local anesthetic spread is indicated in the circled areas. Which nerves are expected to be spared if this is the only injection?

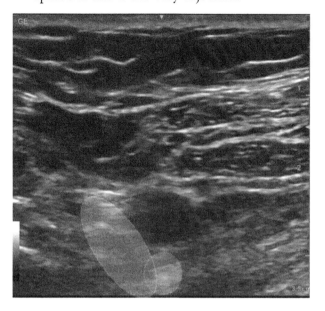

A. Median and radial
B. Ulnar and radial
C. Musculocutaneous and medial antebrachial cutaneous
D. Ulnar, median (partial), medial antebrachial cutaneous, and medial brachial cutaneous

12. A 35-year-old man severed his index and middle fingers in an industrial accident. He is scheduled for urgent reimplantation. The surgeon requests a sympathectomy to the arm over the first postoperative day to improve perfusion. All of the following are viable options EXCEPT:

A. Intravenous regional anesthesia (Bier's block)
B. Infraclavicular block
C. Stellate ganglion block
D. Supraclavicular block

13. A patient is having an infraclavicular catheter placed preoperatively for a distal radius fracture. He is in considerable pain and does not cooperate well during the block, moving around frequently. Imaging the structures of interest is difficult. In the recovery area, he is coughing and complains of shortness of breath. What is the likely diagnosis?

   A. Local anesthetic toxicity

   B. Pneumothorax

   C. Fat embolism

   D. Phrenic nerve injury

14. A patient is receiving an infraclavicular block for elbow arthroplasty. There is a large amount of subcutaneous fat, and the plexus is difficult to visualize. The anesthesiologist attempts to place the needle deep to the axillary artery and begins to inject local anesthetic. The patient winces and complains of sharp pain radiating down the dorsal side of her arm. What is the appropriate action?

   A. Continue injection; this is likely a paresthesia due to pressure from the local anesthetic.

   B. Advance the needle for better positioning.

   C. Ask the patient to take a deep breath.

   D. Withdraw the needle and reassess the needle tip location.

15. A caudal-to-cranial needle path is not recommended for an ultrasound-guided infraclavicular block due to the possibility of encountering which structure?

   A. Lung

   B. Axillary artery

   C. Axillary vein

   D. Subscapular artery

Answers

1. (B) Infraclavicular blocks typically occur at the level of the cords of the brachial plexus. The axillary approach blocks the terminal nerves. The interscalene approach blocks the roots (or trunks), whereas the supraclavicular approach typically blocks the divisions.

2. (C) The infraclavicular approach to the brachial plexus occurs in the axilla. In this space, the subclavian artery has become the axillary artery. The axillary artery lies superior (cephalad) to the axillary vein. In this image, a branch of the axillary artery is noted running superior to the main artery as well.

3. (B) The brachial plexus and axillary vessels lie just deep to the fascia of the pectoralis minor muscle. It is critical to deposit local anesthetic deep to this fascia or the block will fail.

4. (D) The intercostobrachial nerve arises from T2 and is not anesthetized by any approach to the brachial plexus. It may be blocked by subcutaneous infiltration of local anesthetic under the ventral side of the proximal arm.

5. (D) The cords of the brachial plexus surround the axillary artery. With the left side of the screen oriented cephalad, the lateral, posterior, and medial cords are often found at 9 to 10 o'clock, 6 to 7 o'clock, and 4 to 5 o'clock relative to the artery, respectively.

6. (C) The patient most likely had sufficient local anesthetic spread from the initial bolus of local anesthetic. With resolution of the initial block, the lateral cord was not adequately blocked by the infusion, leading to pain in the musculocutaneous nerve distribution.

7. (D) The infraclavicular approach has many advantages, including single needle entry and the included block of the medial brachial cutaneous and medial antebrachial cutaneous nerves. It is also a good location for catheter placement. Needle visualization by ultrasound, however, is often more difficult due to the steep angle of the needle and the depth of the plexus.

8. (A) The axillary vessels and the brachial plexus often lie deep to the clavicle. Abducting the arm and flexing the elbow will often bring the structures caudally, allowing ultrasound visualization. More medial approaches are not recommended due to proximity to the pleura.

9. (C) The local anesthetic is being injected at approximately the 3 o'clock position relative to the axillary artery. The posterior cord lies immediately posterior (6 o'clock) to the axillary artery, and the lateral cord lies at approximately 10 o'clock in this case. The medial cord is at 3 o'clock.

10. (C) Hydrodissection (injection of water or normal saline) is a useful tool to visualize the needle location. Local anesthetic, however, should NOT be injected blindly. Observing tissue movement, choosing an echogenic needle, and manipulating the transducer are all viable options to improve needle visualization.

11. **(D)**   In the image, the medial cord is not in contact with any local anesthetic; hence, any terminal nerves arising from this cord will likely be spared. The medial cord gives rise to the ulnar, part of the median, medial brachial cutaneous, and medial antebrachial cutaneous nerves. The radial nerve arises from the posterior cord, whereas the musculocutaneous nerve arises from the lateral cord.

12. **(A)**   The sympathetic nerves to the arm travel with the peripheral nerves, so any brachial plexus block that would provide anesthesia to the hand will also cause sympathectomy. Intravenous regional anesthesia would not be appropriate for this procedure due to its short duration of action. Although it would not provide analgesia for the surgery, stellate ganglion block would block sympathetic innervation to the arm (as well as the head).

13. **(B)**   Pneumothorax is a possible complication of infraclavicular blocks, particularly if the needle is not continuously visualized or if the patient moves during the procedure. The likelihood of this complication increases as the block location moves proximally along the plexus. Local anesthetic toxicity would present with neurologic and/or cardiac findings. Fat embolism is possible but much less likely. Phrenic nerve injury is very unlikely given the distance between the infraclavicular approach and the phrenic nerve.

14. **(D)**   Sharp, radiating pain is highly suggestive of intraneural injection of local anesthetic. In this case, the pain is in a radial nerve distribution, suggesting needle placement within the posterior cord. The needle should be withdrawn (not advanced) and imaging should be optimized.

15. **(C)**   The axillary vein typically lies inferior (caudal) to the axillary artery. It is commonly difficult to visualize in an upright patient due to collapse. Needle approaches from between the clavicle and axillary artery are unlikely to encounter the vein. Approaching from below, however, runs the risk of transfixing the vein or intravascular injection of local anesthetic.

CHAPTER 7

Suprascapular Nerve Block

Wael Ali Sakr Esa

Questions

DIRECTIONS (Questions 1 and 2): Please match the structure below with the letter that corresponds to it in the ultrasound image.

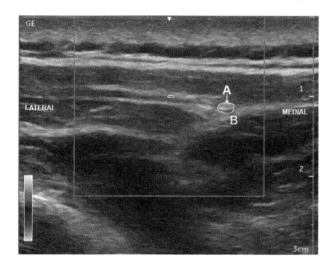

1. Suprascapular artery _____

2. Suprascapular nerve _____

3. All the following statements about a suprascapular nerve block are true EXCEPT:

   A. The suprascapular nerve innervates the supraspinatus and infraspinatus muscles.
   B. The suprascapular nerve provides minimal sensory innervation to the shoulder joint.
   C. The suprascapular nerve originates from the ventral rami of the fifth and sixth cervical nerve roots.
   D. A blockade is performed at the floor of the suprascapular fossa where the suprascapular nerve is covered by the supraspinatus fascia.
   E. Suprascapular nerve blockade is effective for pain control following arthroscopic shoulder surgery.

4. All the following statements about suprascapular nerve block are true EXCEPT:

   A. The suprascapular nerve arises from the C7 and C8 nerve roots.
   B. The suprascapular nerve emerges from the superior trunk of the brachial plexus block.
   C. With the application of colored Doppler, the suprascapular nerve can be visualized medial to the pulsation of the suprascapular artery.
   D. Under ultrasound, the suprascapular nerve is oval or round in shape and slightly hyperechoic structure.

5. A suprascapular nerve block can be used to control pain in the following EXCEPT:

   A. Frozen shoulder
   B. Dislocated shoulder
   C. Rotator cuff syndrome
   D. Fracture humerus
   E. Scapular fracture

6. All of the following statements about a suprascapular nerve block are true EXCEPT:

   A. High-frequency ultrasound probe is preferred to better visualize the nerve and artery
   B. Using color Doppler is helpful as the suprascapular nerve usually lies medial to the suprascapular artery.
   C. The block is not painful to the patient.
   D. Always use echogenic needles as visualization of the needle is difficult due to the steep angle used in performing the block.
   E. The incidence of pneumothorax is very low when performing the block.

Answers

1. Suprascapular artery __A__

2. Suprascapular nerve __B__

3. (B) The suprascapular nerve provides 70% of the sensory innervation to the shoulder. It provides major sensory innervation to the posterior and superior aspects of the shoulder. It is an effective modality for pain control following arthroscopic shoulder surgery. An interscalene brachial plexus block is superior to a suprascapular nerve block in providing pain control following shoulder surgery.

4. (A) The suprascapular nerve arises from the C5 and C6 nerve roots, emerges from the superior trunk of the brachial plexus, and then enters the supraspinatus fossa via the suprascapular notch underneath the superior transverse ligament.

5. (D) The suprascapular nerve innervates up to 70% of the superior and posterior part of the shoulder. The superior articular branch from the suprascapular nerve supplies the coracohumeral ligament, subacromial bursa, and posterior aspect of the acromioclavicular joint capsule, whereas the inferior articular branch from the suprascapular nerve supplies the posterior joint capsule. The suprascapular nerve has no innervation to the anterior and inferior shoulder regions.

6. (C) The block is painful as the needle will pass through muscles, so prepare your patient with local anesthesia, midazolam, and fentanyl. The incidence of pneumothorax associated with a suprascapular nerve block is reported as less than 1%. The use of ultrasound and an in-plane approach will decrease this risk markedly.

CHAPTER 8

Neuraxial Anesthesia

Maria Bauer

Questions

1. The risk of iatrogenic spinal cord trauma can be completely eliminated by:

   A. Needle placement through the L3 to L4 vertebral interspace

   B. Expecting resistance prior to entering the epidural space during midline approach to the neuraxis

   C. Expecting uniform dorsoventral dimension of the posterior epidural space along the entire vertebral column

   D. None of the above

2. Spinal cord perfusion pressure can potentially be diminished by all of the following EXCEPT:

   A. An increased systemic to cerebrospinal fluid pressure gradient

   B. Excessive volumes of local anesthetics

   C. Chronic morphine administration via intrathecal delivery systems

   D. Surgical procedures performed in extreme lateral flexion in patients with severe spinal stenosis

3. A needle directed too medially to the facet within the lateral recess may impede flow through the:

   A. Anterior spinal artery

   B. Posterior spinal artery

   C. Spinal branch of the segmental artery at the dorsal nerve root

   D. Central artery

4. In a morbidly obese patient with known extradural tumor at the T7 vertebral level, awaiting thoracotomy for pneumonectomy:

   A. Radiologic evaluation of the neuraxis should be considered to better characterize the extent of the tumor.

   B. Epidural catheter placement and bolusing local anesthetic via the catheter can always be safely performed.

   C. Significant and prolonged systemic hypotension is preferred to minimize blood loss.

   D. Surgical positioning is not relevant as long as it provides excellent exposure of the operative field.

5. Which of the following is associated with an increased risk of complications after neuraxial blockade?

   A. Hypertrophy of the ligamentum flavum

   B. Nonneutral patient positioning

   C. Surface landmarks that are difficult to appreciate

   D. All of the above

6. Which of the following statements regarding neuraxial anesthesia and obstructive spinal pathology is true?

   A. When epidural anesthesia is complicated by development of an epidural hematoma, patients with severe spinal stenosis are more likely to experience severe postoperative complications.

   B. When neuraxial anesthesia is planned, increasing the volume of local anesthetic is recommended to achieve adequate segmental spread.

   C. When neuraxial anesthesia is planned, reducing the total mass (volume × concentration) of the local anesthetic is not recommended as this may increase the risk of local anesthetic toxicity.

   D. Asymptomatic patients do not have spinal stenosis; therefore, neuraxial techniques can be performed without the risk of adverse outcomes.

7. In normotensive, unanesthetized adults, the lower limit of spinal cord autoregulation is approximately:

   A. 50 to 55 mm Hg
   B. 55 to 60 mm Hg
   C. 60 to 65 mm Hg
   D. 65 to 70 mm Hg

8. Which of the following statements regarding spinal cord perfusion is true?

   A. Preoperative hypertension is an accurate predictor of the lower limit of spinal cord autoregulation.

   B. Intrathecal epinephrine adversely affects the spinal cord blood flow.

   C. Sickle cell disease may increase the risk of spinal cord ischemia.

   D. Prolonged sensory and motor blockade after neuraxial anesthesia or analgesia is a sign of residual local anesthetic effect; therefore, no further workup is necessary.

9. The cauda equina is particularly vulnerable to local anesthetic toxicity because the neural elements:

   A. Are not fully protected by myelin
   B. May have limited cerebrospinal fluid (CSF) dilutional capacity
   C. May have reduced drug clearance
   D. All of the above

10. Which of the following is most likely a risk factor of cauda equina syndrome (CES)?

    A. African descent
    B. Disk herniation
    C. 2% chloroprocaine
    D. Female gender

11. Twenty-four hours after a hemorrhoidectomy, a 54-year-old obese patient with history of diabetes develops low back pain, aching in his buttocks and posterior thighs, and pinprick sensation in the plantar aspect of his feet. Upon review of the anesthetic record, it appears that he received an atraumatic spinal anesthetic with 45 mg 1.5% mepivacaine through the L3 to L4 vertebral interspace. The surgery lasted 1 hour and was performed in the jackknife position. There was no evidence of hemodynamic instability or adverse drug reaction. On initial assessment, the patient is afebrile, and vital signs are within normal limits. Physical examination reveals preserved motor and sensory function. Spinal MRI ruled out infection, trauma, and disk disease. Which of the following is most likely to be the most helpful in the subsequent management of this patient?

    A. Order electromyoneurography to rule out denervation injury.

    B. Schedule the patient for epidural steroid injection after a trial of gabapentin and tricyclic antidepressants.

    C. Reassure the patient and treat with NSAIDs until symptoms resolve.

    D. Order a neurosurgical consultation for immediate surgical management of CES.

12. Regarding the safety of performing a neuraxial blockade on patients taking oral anticoagulants, which of the following statements is INCORRECT?

A. Dabigatran should be discontinued at least 48 hours before neuraxial injection.

B. Prasugrel should be discontinued at least 7 to 10 days before neuraxial injection.

C. In patients taking fondaparinux, if neuraxial technique has to be performed, single needle neuraxial technique is recommended, and an indwelling catheter placement should be avoided.

D. In patients on recent bivalirudin therapy, anticoagulant effect should be pharmacologically reversed prior to performance of neuraxial techniques.

13. Regarding the safety of neuraxial anesthesia in patients taking oral anticoagulants, which of the following statement is FALSE?

A. It is safe to perform a neuraxial block on patients taking aspirin and multiple nonaspirin NSAIDs, as long as discontinuation is based on each drug's specific half-life.

B. Prasugrel should be stopped 7 to 10 days before a neuraxial injection.

C. Fresh frozen plasma is effective in the reversal of dabigatran.

D. In patients at high risk for angina, epidural catheters can be removed safely, and neuraxial injections can be performed 5 days after clopidogrel is discontinued.

14. Select the correct statement.

A. Spinal anesthesia may be safely performed in patients with evidence of systemic infection and appropriate response to antimicrobial therapy.

B. In patients with evidence of systemic infection, placement of an indwelling neuraxial catheter has not been shown to increase the risk of infectious complications.

C. Routine use of preprocedural antibiotics reduces the risk of infection in patients with no evidence of systemic infection.

D. Spinal anesthesia for procedures associated with transient bacteremia is contraindicated.

15. The risk of arachnoiditis resulting from the use of chlorhexidine as a skin disinfectant is minimal when:

A. Chlorhexidine is allowed to completely dry on the skin before needle placement.

B. There is temporal and physical separation of block tray from chlorhexidine.

C. Care is taken to avoid needle or catheter contamination from chlorhexidine.

D. All of the above

16. Which of the following is NOT the risk factor of spontaneous spinal hematoma formation in patients receiving antithrombotic therapy?

A. Increased age

B. Concomitant aspirin use

C. International normalized ratio (INR) of 2.0

D. Thrombolytic therapy

17. The risk of spinal hematoma formation, relative to patients with no preexisting coagulopathy and atraumatic needle placement, is the greatest in patients:

    A. With no preexisting coagulopathy after traumatic needle placement

    B. Receiving heparin longer than 1hour after atraumatic needle placement

    C. On aspirin, receiving heparin longer than 1 hour after needle placement

    D. On heparin anticoagulation longer than 1 hour after traumatic needle placement

18. Following an epidural catheter placement, a patient develops fever, headache, and meningeal signs. Lower extremity reflexes are diminished. Spinal imaging reveals fluid collection at the L3 to L4 intervertebral space. Which of the following statements regarding the most likely diagnosis is true?

    A. Diagnosis is confirmed with lumbar puncture, so a lumbar puncture should always be performed.

    B. Mortality is less than 5% if appropriate antibiotic treatment is initiated.

    C. The most sensitive diagnostic modality for evaluation is spinal MRI.

    D. The best chance of neurological recovery is achieved with initiation of targeted antibiotic therapy and surgical intervention after culture results become available.

19. Risk factors associated with an increased risk of development of infected epidural fluid collection include:

    A. The use of pharmacologic thromboprophylaxis

    B. Longer catheter time in situ

    C. HIV

    D. All of the above

20. Muscle spasm after the resolution of an epidural block is most likely due to:

    A. Methylparaben

    B. EDTA

    C. Metabisulfite

    D. Epinephrine

21. In sensitive individuals, rash, urticaria, potential airway obstruction, and anaphylaxis are more likely to be observed in all of the following EXCEPT:

    A. Bupivacaine with methylparaben

    B. 2-chloroprocaine with EDTA

    C. Ropivacaine

    D. Tetracaine

22. When administered intrathecally, clonidine provides analgesic effect by:

    A. Binding to α_2 receptors in the substantia gelatinosa in the spinal cord

    B. Binding to the intermediolateral column in the spinal cord

    C. Interacting with excitatory AMPA and inhibitory GABA receptors

    D. All of the above

23. All of the following are recognized risk factors for spinal cord infarction EXCEPT:

    A. Hypotension 10% to 15% below baseline mean arterial pressure for 20 minutes or longer

    B. Hypotension 20% to 30% below baseline mean arterial pressure for 20 minutes or longer

    C. History of tobacco use

    D. History of vascular disease

24. Which of the following will most likely decrease the risk of developing CES after a spinal anesthetic?

  A. Redosing of subarachnoid local anesthetic if maldistribution of the local anesthetic within the intrathecal space is suspected

  B. Avoidance of supranormal doses of intrathecal local anesthetic in the setting of a failed spinal anesthetic

  C. Using hyperbaric 5% lidocaine for a single-injection spinal anesthetic to ensure appropriate subarachnoidal spread

  D. Insertion of a small gauge intrathecal catheter instead of performing a single-injection subarachnoid block for surgical anesthesia in patients with known severe spinal stenosis at the level of the intended injection

25. The incidence of postdural puncture headache decreases with:

  A. Decreasing age

  B. Increasing age

  C. Needle insertion perpendicular to the dural fibers

  D. Identifying the epidural space by the loss of resistance to air as opposed to loss of resistance to saline technique

26. The absolute contraindication to spinal anesthesia is:

  A. Preexisting sensorimotor neuropathy

  B. Chorioamnionitis

  C. Patient refusal

  D. Unknown duration of surgery

27. Hemodynamic changes produced by high epidural anesthesia without epinephrine added to the local anesthetic solution include:

  A. Increased stroke volume, decreased total peripheral resistance, unchanged cardiac output, and unchanged arterial pressure

  B. Decreased stroke volume, increased total peripheral resistance, unchanged cardiac output, and unchanged arterial pressure

  C. Decreased stroke volume, decreased total peripheral resistance, decreased cardiac output, and decreased arterial pressure

  D. Increased stroke volume, increased peripheral resistance, increased cardiac output, and increased arterial pressure

28. Hemodynamic changes produced by high epidural anesthesia with epinephrine added to the local anesthetic solution include:

  A. Decreased stroke volume, decreased total peripheral resistance, decreased cardiac output, and decreased arterial pressure

  B. Increased stroke volume, increased total peripheral resistance, increased cardiac output, and increased arterial pressure

  C. Increased stroke volume, decreased total peripheral resistance, increased cardiac output, and decreased arterial pressure

  D. Decreased stroke volume, increased peripheral resistance, decreased cardiac output, and increased arterial pressure

29. Regarding the blood supply of the spinal cord and cauda equina, which of the following is true?

   A. The spinal cord and the cauda equina receive two-thirds of their blood supply from the posterior spinal artery.

   B. The artery supplying two-thirds of the spinal cord and cauda equina can be directly injured from the midline or paramedian approach during placement of an epidural catheter.

   C. Damage to the posterior blood supply of the spinal cord is mitigated by the redundancy of the posterior spinal artery system.

   D. The risk of injury to a radicular artery subsequently, resulting in secondary spinal cord damage during transforaminal procedures, is negligible due to the redundancy of the arterial supply to radicular branches.

30. Regarding neuraxial techniques in patients under deep sedation, which of the following statements is FALSE?

   A. Deep sedation in an adult removes any ability for the patient to recognize and report warning signs that may herald needle contact with the spinal cord.

   B. Deep sedation in a child enhances cooperation and immobility, a benefit that likely outweighs the risk of removing any ability for the patient to report warning signs that may herald needle contact with the spinal cord.

   C. The use of ultrasound during neuraxial anesthesia will reliably prevent needle contact with the spinal cord in adults under deep sedation.

   D. To minimize complications, neuraxial anesthesia or interventional pain procedures should rarely be performed in adult patients with compromised sensorium.

Answers

1. **(D)** The incidence of iatrogenic direct needle- or catheter-related injury to the spinal cord is unknown but is reported to be distinctly rare. Iatrogenic direct mechanical injuries occur by several mechanisms and have been attributed to basic anatomic characteristics of the neuraxis. First, although the termination of the conus medullaris has been commonly described as terminating in the L1 to L2 interspace in adults, its terminus has been found to vary between interspace T12 to L4. Inaccurate identification of a vertebral level during performance of neuraxial anesthesia, especially in patients with obesity, kyphoscoliosis, or previous spinal surgery, further contributes to direct needle- and catheter-related spinal cord injury. Second, there may be an incomplete posterior midline fusion of the ligamentum flavum, failing to provide the abrupt change in tissue density that clinicians utilize when using the loss-of-resistance technique. Third, there is a progressive narrowing of the posterior epidural space from caudad (5 to 13 mm in the lumbar region) to cephalad (2 to 4 mm at the low thoracic, 1 to 2 mm at the high thoracic, and 0.4 mm at the cervical levels); therefore, the margin for error during needle advancement varies at different vertebral levels.

2. **(A)** Indirect spinal cord injury may result from conditions leading to diminished spinal cord perfusion sufficient enough to cause ischemia. Spinal cord perfusion pressure (SCPP) is determined by the pressure gradient between the systemic mean arterial pressure (MAP) and the CSF pressure (SCPP=MAP−CSF pressure). SCPP becomes compromised when there is insufficient arterial inflow, inhibited venous outflow, or elevated CSF pressure within the neuraxis. Significant and prolonged systemic hypotension lowers SCPP if CSF pressure is unchanged or elevated. Space-occupying lesions (such as epidural hematoma, abscess, or excessive accumulation of local anesthetics), spinal stenosis, or intradural or extradural masses (such as granulomas that form at the tip of implanted intrathecal catheters) may either exert direct compression on the spinal cord or increase the intrathecal or epidural pressure.

3. **(C)** See Figures 10-2 and 10-3 in: Neal JM, Rathmell JP. *Complications in regional anesthesia and pain medicine*, 2nd ed. Philadelphia: Lippincott Williams & Wilkins, 2013, pp 118–119.

4. **(A)** In patients with space-occupying neuraxial lesion, near the level of a planned epidural injection, radiologic evaluation of the neuraxis should be considered to better characterize the extent of the mass. Such lesions have been associated with temporary or permanent neurologic deficit due to inadequate neural blood flow, especially when they coexist with epidural space-occupying lesions or processes, such as fluid accumulation within the epidural space. Spinal cord perfusion pressure can be further compromised by prolonged hypoperfusion or certain surgical positions such as flexed lateral decubitus position.

5. **(D)** Misidentification of the vertebral level, unrecognized lateral needle placement, challenging surface anatomy, disease processes that decrease the cross-sectional area within the spinal canal, and factors that compromise spinal cord perfusion pressure have all been associated with adverse neurological outcomes after spinal and epidural anesthetic techniques.

6. (A) Any condition or disease process that decreases the cross-section area of the space inside the vertebral canal makes patients prone to impaired spinal cord perfusion, especially with concomitant mass effect within the spinal canal. Patients with severe spinal stenosis may be more likely to have more severe postoperative neurologic deficits when a neuraxial anesthetic is complicated by development of hematoma or abscess. Increasing the volume or concentration of a local anesthetic may result in unnecessarily extensive segmental spread of the local anesthetic and increased risk of local anesthetic toxicity. Symptoms do not always correlate with the severity of disease as even moderately severe spinal stenosis may remain asymptomatic.

7. (C) Recent studies have found that the lower limit of cerebral and spinal autoregulation in normotensive, unanesthetized adults with intact blood-neural tissue barrier is 60 to 65 mm Hg, higher than the previously accepted MAP range of 50 to 60 mm Hg. There is an existing physiologic reserve that affords some degree of protection during periods of hypoperfusion, which may be significantly compromised by the presence of unrecognized hypertension, increased local tissue pressure, abnormal vascular anatomy, low flow states, disruption of the blood-neural tissue barrier, and/or impaired O_2 carrying capacity, such as in anemia or erythrocyte sludging.

8. (C) Preexisting hypertension appears to be a poor predictor of the lower limit of autoregulation, except when systolic pressure is greater than 160 mm Hg. The use of intrathecal or intravenous epinephrine or phenylephrine has not been conclusively shown to have any adverse effects on spinal cord blood flow. Any conditions associated with impaired O_2 carrying capacity and/or erythrocyte sludging, such as anemia or sickle cell disease, may increase the risk of injury during and after neuraxial anesthesia. In any instance, when a neuraxial technique is followed by an unexpectedly long period of recovery, nonresolving motor weakness, numbness, or block extending beyond the distribution of the intended procedure, reversible causes must be ruled out by reducing or discontinuing local anesthetic infusion, reassessment of the patient within an hour, and ordering the appropriate imaging, preferably MRI, to rule out compressive lesion or spinal cord ischemia. Neurologic consultation is recommended to help evaluate the nature and mechanisms of insults and coordinate further management.

9. (D) Local anesthetic-induced neurotoxicity may have an enhanced effect on the cauda equina due to the large surface area afforded by the long nerve roots that have only partial or absent myelin covering, relative hypovascularity, and limited CSF dilutional capacity when local anesthetic is injected into the dural root sleeve.

10. (B) Individuals with disk herniation are most at risk for developing CES. Race does not appear to have a role; however, individuals of African descent appear to have the least risk of developing CES. Males are at slightly increased risk as compared with females. There is no sufficient evidence to determine the risk of CES with 2% chloroprocaine.

11. (C) Transient neurologic symptoms (TNS) may be observed with any local anesthetic; however, the relative risk of TNS is 1 to 7 when lidocaine or mepivacaine is used and seven times that of bupivacaine, prilocaine, or procaine. Classically, symptoms present within 24 hours after the resolution of spinal anesthesia. TNS may manifest as low back pain and/or unilateral or bilateral buttock pain that may or may not radiate to the anterior and posterior thighs. TNS is not associated with loss of reflexes, sensory function, or sphincter tone. There are no abnormal radiologic findings. Symptoms typically resolve within 6 hours to 4 days from onset and respond well to NSAIDs. In the absence of other neurologic deficits, no further workup, treatment, or consulting surgical services is warranted.

12. (D) According to the most recent guidelines for antithrombotic therapy from the American Society of Regional Anesthesia and Pain Medicine (ASRA), dabigatran should be discontinued at least 48 hours before neuraxial injection. Prasugrel should be discontinued at least 7 to 10 days before neuraxial injection. In patients taking fondaparinux, if neuraxial technique has to be performed, single-needle neuraxial technique is recommended, and indwelling catheter placement should be avoided. Recombinant hirudin derivatives are used in cases of heparin-induced thrombocytopenia or as an adjunct when percutaneous angioplasty is performed. The anticoagulant effect of recombinant hirudin derivatives (for example, bivalirudin, lepirudin, desirudin) is present for up to 3 hours after discontinuation of their infusion and cannot be pharmacologically reversed. The most recent ASRA guidelines recommend against neuraxial anesthesia in patients on recent recombinant hirudin derivative therapy.

13. (C) Dabigatran etexilate is a specific and reversible inhibitor of both free and clot-bound thrombin. When taken by mouth, it is absorbed from the gastrointestinal tract as a prodrug and is converted into dabigatran, its active form. Eighty percent of dabigatran is excreted by the kidneys without further metabolism. Its anticoagulant effect at therapeutic concentrations is most reliably monitored by thrombin time and ecarin clotting time (ECT) and cannot be offset by administration of fresh frozen plasma. Reversal of the anticoagulant effect can theoretically be achieved by administering recombinant factor VII. For patients with significant bleeding due to dabigatran, dialysis should be considered. Dabigatran should be discontinued 7 days prior to a planned procedure. For shorter periods, normal thrombin time should be documented. The first postoperative dose should be given no earlier than 24 hours after needle placement. Neuraxial catheters should be removed at least 2 hours prior to the initiation of dabigatran therapy.

14. (A) Available data suggests that spinal anesthesia may be safely performed in patients with evidence of systemic infection and appropriate response to antibiotic treatment. Epidural catheter placement in the same patient population is associated with an increased risk of infectious complications. Spinal anesthesia may be safely performed in patients at risk for low-grade transient bacteremia. Patients with untreated systemic infection should not receive neuraxial anesthetic. Routine use of prophylactic antibiotics before performing neuraxial anesthesia in patients without evidence of infection is not recommended.

15. (D) Arachnoiditis is a diffuse inflammatory reaction of the meninges associated most commonly with nonanesthetic conditions, such as trauma, infection, contrast media, or multiple back surgeries. The incidence of arachnoiditis directly stemming from neuraxial techniques is extremely rare. Chlorhexidine has been found to be superior to povidone-iodine as a disinfectant agent, and its use as an antiseptic of choice before neuraxial techniques is now recommended. According to the ASRA Practice Advisory on Neurologic Injuries, to reduce the risk of chemical arachnoiditis due to skin disinfectants, chlorhexidine/alcohol mixtures should be allowed to fully dry before needle placement, complete physical and temporal separation of disinfectant from the procedural tray should be maintained, and care should be taken to avoid needle or catheter contamination from disinfectant spraying or dripping.

16. (C) Neuraxial hematomas are rare complications of spinal and epidural anesthetics, resulting in potentially permanent neurological damage. The overall incidence is approximated to be 1.9 in 150,000 to 200,000 neuraxial anesthetics. In the absence of traumatic needle placement, spinal hematomas may occur spontaneously in patients receiving antithrombotic or antiplatelet therapy. Risk factors include increased age; female gender; concomitant aspirin use; history of gastrointestinal bleeding; and the intensity and length of anticoagulant or antiplatelet therapy. An INR of 2.0 to 3.0 is associated with a low risk of bleeding. Thrombolytic therapy poses the greatest risk of bleeding complications. (From: Neal JM, Rathmell JP. *Complications in regional anesthesia and pain medicine*, 2nd ed. Philadelphia: Lippincott Williams & Wilkins, 2013, Chapter 4: Bleeding complications.)

17. (D) Patient characteristics and anesthetic variables are risk modifiers of serious hemorrhagic complications of neuraxial anesthetics. Compared with an atraumatic needle placement in a patient with no preexisting coagulopathy (relative risk [RR]: 1.0), the risk of serious bleeding complications is the greatest in instances of traumatic needle placement (RR=112), followed by heparin anticoagulation with concomitant aspirin use (RR=26), and traumatic needle placement in patients with no preexisting coagulopathy (RR=11.2). The relative risk of spinal hematoma in patients receiving heparin more than 1 hour after atraumatic needle placement is 2.18 compared with patients not on heparin anticoagulation.

18. (C) Bacterial meningitis is a medical emergency carrying a 30% mortality rate even with appropriate, aggressive antibiotic therapy, initiated without delay. The diagnosis is typically confirmed with lumbar puncture. If epidural abscess is suspected or present, lumbar puncture should be avoided as the procedure would increase the risk of intrathecal contamination. The most sensitive diagnostic modality for suspected infectious processes is MRI; however, CT scanning and myelography can be alternatives to MRI if it is unable to be performed. Early surgical intervention (within 12 hours) offers the best chance of neurologic recovery. A delay in diagnosis and treatment even a few hours significantly worsens neurologic outcome.

19. (D) The following factors have been implicated in the development of infectious neuraxial complications after spinal or epidural anesthesia: indwelling epidural catheter (versus spinal anesthetic); prolonged duration of the catheter in situ; immunocompromised or chronically ill patient; local infection at the insertion site; abandoning strict adherence to aseptic techniques; and thromboprophylaxis.

20. (B) Back pain after the resolution of an epidural block is most likely due to calcium-chelator EDTA. Although not a common additive, it has been observed that EDTA, substituting metabisulfite as antioxidant in 2-chloroprocaine solutions, produced paraspinal muscle spasm upon resolution of the epidural block. Methylparabens, used as antibacterials in local anesthetic solutions, are metabolized to para-aminobenzoic acid (PABA) that may trigger true allergic reactions in sensitive individuals. Metabisulfite is added to vasoconstrictor-containing solutions to prevent oxidative biodegradation and has been reported to induce a range of adverse clinical effects, ranging from dermatitis, urticaria, flushing, hypotension, abdominal pain, and diarrhea to life-threatening bronchospasm and anaphylactic reactions. Epinephrine has not been shown to cause muscle spasm and is the mainstay in the treatment of adverse drug reactions leading to severe cardiovascular and respiratory compromise.

21. (C) Ester-type local anesthetics (for example, procaine, chloroprocaine, and tetracaine) are associated with a higher incidence of hypersensitivity reactions due to their metabolism to PABA. PABA is also a metabolite of parabens, commonly used as preservatives in cosmetic and pharmaceutical products. Amide local anesthetics (for example, lidocaine, mepivacaine, bupivacaine, or ropivacaine) do not undergo metabolism to PABA, and therefore, hypersensitivity to amide local anesthetics is rare. Ropivacaine is merchandised as a preservative-free solution; mounting a true allergic response to its use is therefore extremely unlikely.

22. (D) When administered intrathecally, clonidine, a centrally acting α_2-receptor agonist, provides analgesic effect by binding to α_2 receptors in the substantia gelatinosa in the spinal cord, binding to the intermediolateral column in the spinal cord, and interacting with excitatory AMPA and inhibitory GABA receptors, with resultant inhibition of substance P release and firing of wide dynamic range neurons in the dorsal horn of the spinal cord. Peripherally, it appears to act more like a local anesthetic. With doses between 30 and 300 mcg, clonidine predictably and reliably prolongs the duration of sensory and motor block without having a significant effect on the onset of block. Systemic side effects are hypotension, sedation, and dry mouth. No toxicity was reported with clonidine when administered intrathecally up to 300 mcg.

23. (A) Perioperative spinal cord ischemia is an extremely rare event, most often associated with cardiac, aortic, or spine surgeries. Insults to the spinal cord, sufficient to cause ischemia or infarction, imply either mechanical injury to the spinal vasculature, an embolic event, or tissue hypoperfusion. Recent data suggest that the lower limit of cerebral and spinal autoregulation (LLA) is likely higher than previously thought. Current recommendations emphasize the importance of avoiding prolonged (especially 20 minutes or longer) hypotension (greater than 20% to 30% below baseline mean arterial pressure) during neuraxial anesthetics. Other recognized risk factors are those recognized for vascular disease: diabetes, tobacco use, obesity, increasing age, hypertension, hypercholesterolemia, and high levels of homocysteine. It is recommended that "anesthesiologists strive to maintain blood pressure within 20% to 30% of baseline and that persistent hypotension be treated."

24. **(B)** CES is a medical/surgical emergency secondary to diffuse injury to the nerve roots distal to the conus medullaris. Manifesting signs and symptoms may include severe low back pain, anesthesia or paresthesia involving the S3 to S5 dermatomes, decreased urinary and anal sphincter tone, decreased urinary detrusor tone, unilateral or bilateral lower extremity sensory loss, weakness or paraplegia, and sexual dysfunction. Factors that may increase the risk of developing CES are moderate to severe spinal stenosis, degenerative disk disease, a history of prior back surgery, certain congenital spinal abnormalities (for example, spina bifida, lesions, or tumors affecting the spinal canal), aberrant spinal vasculature, needle trauma, infection or hemorrhage, or nonneutral positions during the perioperative period. Local anesthetics in clinically appropriate doses have been implicated as a cause of CES following spinal anesthesia. Hyperbaric solutions injected through small-bore catheters (microcatheters) have been shown to produce poor mixture within the cerebrospinal fluid, resulting in accumulation of toxic local anesthetic concentrations around the cauda equina nerve roots. Known anesthetic-related risk factors are supranormal doses of intrathecal local anesthetics (that is, redosing a failed or partial spinal anesthetic), maldistribution of local anesthetics within the subarachnoidal space, or the use of small-bore intrathecal catheters. It is advised to carefully weigh the risks to benefits of subarachnoidal block in patients with known moderate to severe spinal stenosis.

25. **(B)** Postdural puncture headache (PDPH) is a common complication of neuraxial anesthesia. The risk of PDPH was found to be lower with epidural anesthesia but may occur in up to 50% in the cases of accidental dural puncture with large-bore epidural needles. PDPH is a characteristically positional, fronto-occipital headache, believed to result from CSF loss through the meningeal needle hole. The incidence of PDPH decreases with increasing age and the use of small-diameter noncutting spinal needles. Inserting cutting needles perpendicular to dural fibers under longitudinal tension is thought to produce a slit-like dural hole that will pull open under the longitudinal tension of the spinal dura mater. The use of fluid, instead of air, for localizing the epidural space during attempted epidural anesthesia has not been shown to modify the risk of accidental dural puncture but has been shown to decrease the risk of subsequent PDPH.

26. **(C)** The absolute contraindications to spinal anesthetics are patient refusal, severe hypovolemia, uncorrected coagulopathy, infection at the site of injection, and increased intracranial pressure. Infection distant to the site of injection and appropriately treated with antibiotics, preexisting neurologic disease, or unknown duration of surgery are not con-

sidered as absolute contraindications to spinal anesthesia but may increase risks of complications associated with neuraxial blockade.

27. (C) High epidural block with local anesthetic solutions that do not contain epinephrine will result in decreased stroke volume, decreased total peripheral resistance, decreased cardiac output, and decreased arterial blood pressure.

28. (C) High epidural block with local anesthetic solutions that contain epinephrine will result in a significant increase in stroke volume and cardiac output and decrease in total peripheral vascular resistance and arterial pressure. The decrease in peripheral vascular resistance is attributed to a peripheral β2-receptor effect of low doses of epinephrine resulting in vasodilation and a subsequent decrease in total peripheral vascular resistance, as well as epinephrine-induced venoconstriction, resulting in an increased venous return.

29. (C) The spinal cord and cauda equina receive two-thirds of their blood supply from the anterior spinal artery. The anterior spinal artery cannot be directly injured by posterior midline or paramedian approaches without first traversing the spinal cord. Damage to the posterior circulation is mitigated by the redundancy of the posterior spinal artery system. The segmental or spinal branches, however, may be exposed to needle trauma, especially with lateral deviation or intentional placement of the needle near a segmental artery. Radicular arteries may be one of the few arteries that continue on to become a medullary artery supplying the spinal cord. This is of importance when performing transforaminal procedures, as injury to the radicular artery is a known complication of such techniques.

30. (C) Wakefulness is considered a potentially useful monitoring tool when used during adult neuraxial anesthesia or interventional pain procedures but not during pediatric neuraxial anesthesia or interventional pain procedures. It may alert to direct nerve injury, or other, indirect neuraxial-related complications, such as total spinal anesthesia or local anesthetic systemic toxicity. Warning signs such as paresthesia or pain during injection of local anesthetic inconsistently herald spinal cord injury from needle trauma; however, deep sedation in an adult removes any ability for the patient to recognize and report warning signs that may herald needle contact with the spinal cord. Neuraxial regional anesthesia or interventional pain medicine procedures should be performed rarely in adults whose sensorium is compromised. In pediatric patients, deep sedation does increase cooperation and immobility and likely enhances the safety of neuraxial techniques. Currently, there are no data to support that ultrasound guidance of needle placement during neuraxial anesthesia reduces the risk of neuraxial injury in patients under general anesthesia or deep sedation.

Bibliography

Allergic reactions to Local Anesthetics. Pharmacology Update. Cleveland Clinic Center for Continuing Education. Volume IV, Number 1, January/February 2001. <https://www.clevelandclinicmeded.com/medicalpubs/pharmacy/JanFeb2001/allergicreaction.htm>.

Local anesthetic. Transient neurologic symptoms. <https://www.openanesthesia.org/local_anesthetic_transient_neurologic_symptoms/>.

Narouze, S., Benzon, H.T., et al., 2015. Interventional spine and pain procedures in patients on antiplatelet and anticoagulant medications. Guidelines from the American Society of Regional Anesthesia and Pain Medicine, the European Society of Regional Anesthesia and Pain Therapy, the American Academy of Pain Medicine, the International Neuromodulation Society, the North American Neuromodulation Society, and the World Institute of Pain. Reg. Anesth. Pain Med. 40, 182–212.

Neal, J.M., Barrington, M.J., et al., 2015. The second ASRA practice advisory on neurologic complications associated with regional anesthesia and pain medicine. Executive Summary. Reg. Anesth. Pain Med. 40, 401–430.

Neal, J.M., Kopp, S.L., et al., 2015. Anatomy and pathophysiology of spinal cord injury associated with regional anesthesia and pain medicine. Reg. Anesth. Pain Med. 40, 506–525.

Neal, J.M., Rathmell, J.P., 2013. Complications in Regional Anesthesia and Pain Medicine, second ed. Lippincott Williams & Wilkins, Philadelphia.

Regional Anesthesia in the Anticoagulated Patient. <http://www.nysora.com/mobile/regional-anesthesia/foundations-of-ra/3300-ra-in-anticoagulated-patient.html>.

Vally, H., Misso, N.L., 2012. Adverse reactions to the sulphite additives. Gastroenterol. Hepatol. Bed Bench 5 (1), 16–23.

CHAPTER 9

Femoral Block

John George

Questions

1. In a typical transverse scan of the inguinal region, the femoral nerve is immediately deep to the following structure:

   A. The fascia of the iliopsoas muscle
   B. The fascia iliaca
   C. The fascia lata
   D. The femoral artery

2. The base of the femoral triangle is formed by all of these muscles EXCEPT:

   A. The sartorius muscle
   B. The iliopsoas muscle
   C. The pectineus muscle
   D. The adductor longus muscle

3. All of the following are reliable responses of ensuring success of a femoral nerve block EXCEPT:

   A. A quadriceps muscle twitch
   B. Stimulation of the femoral nerve at 0.4 mA
   C. A sartorius muscle twitch
   D. A patella twitch

4. Which of the following is the best location for ultimate placement of the needle when using ultrasound guidance for a femoral nerve block?

   A. Anterior to the femoral triangle
   B. Posterior to the femoral triangle
   C. Medial aspect of the femoral triangle
   D. Lateral aspect of the femoral triangle

5. All of the following can be used to distinguish the femoral nerve from an inguinal lymph node EXCEPT:

   A. Scanning proximally
   B. Scanning distally
   C. Scanning in the long axis view
   D. Noting a hyperechoic structure

6. Which of the following corresponds to the structure denoted by the arrowheads in the following image?

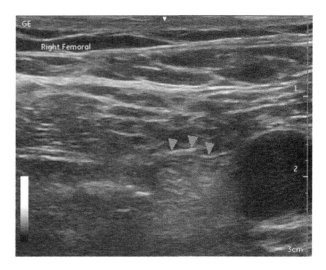

   A. Transversalis fascia
   B. Fascia iliaca
   C. Sartorius muscle fascia
   D. Fascia lata

7. The femoral nerve innervates all of the following EXCEPT:
   A. The gracilis muscle
   B. The vastus lateralis muscle
   C. The pectineus muscle
   D. The hip joint

8. Which of the following represents the MOST ideal ultrasound transducer for performing a femoral nerve block in a 70 kg patient with a normal body mass index?
   A. A curvilinear probe at 2 MHz
   B. A linear probe at 5 MHz
   C. A linear probe at 12 MHz
   D. A curvilinear probe at 5 MHz

9. When considering absolute versus relative contraindications to performance of a femoral nerve block, all of these patients have a relative contraindications EXCEPT:
   A. A patient with an allergy to local anesthetics
   B. A patient with a femoral artery vascular graft
   C. A patient taking Plavix for a drug eluting stent placed 2 years ago
   D. A patient with diabetic neuropathy involving the surgical extremity

10. A femoral nerve block can be used as an adjunct to control pain in each of these surgeries EXCEPT:
    A. Proximal femur surgery
    B. Knee surgery
    C. Medial foot surgery
    D. Proximal anterior thigh surgery

11. Which of the following corresponds to the structure denoted by the arrowhead in the following image?

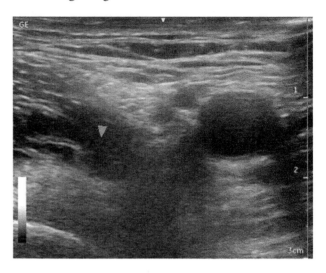

   A. Air artifact
   B. The femoral nerve
   C. The iliopsoas muscle
   D. Femoral nerve acoustic shadowing

12. In general, the depth setting on the ultrasound that optimizes image quality is:
    A. Less than 2 cm
    B. 2 to 3 cm
    C. 3 to 4 cm
    D. 4 to 7 cm

Answers

1. (B) While all the structures can be found in a typical transverse scan of the inguinal region, the femoral nerve is typically superficial to the iliopsoas muscle and lateral to the femoral artery. The fascia lata is superficial and can be found in the subcutaneous layer.

2. (A) Posteriorly, the base of the femoral triangle is formed by the pectineus, iliopsoas, and adductor longus muscles. Part of the adductor longus muscle also forms the medial border of the triangle, while the superior and lateral borders are formed by the inguinal ligament and medial border of the sartorius muscle, respectively.

3. (C) A twitch of the sartorius muscle can be commonly seen when using nerve stimulation for localization of the femoral nerve. A band-like contraction of the thigh without movement of the patella is often how sartorius muscle stimulation manifests and why it can be mistaken for stimulation of the femoral nerve. Sartorius muscle stimulation is not a reliable response because the nerve branches to the sartorius muscle off of the femoral nerve may be outside of the femoral sheath.

4. (D) The posterior division of the femoral nerve innervates the quadriceps muscle and is commonly found on the lateral aspect of the femoral triangle. Correspondingly, the goal of needle tip placement is immediately adjacent to the lateral aspect of the femoral nerve with confirmation of local anesthetic deposition visualized by lifting of the femoral nerve off the iliopsoas muscle surface or by the spread of the local anesthetic immediately above the nerve in the wedge-shaped space lateral to the femoral artery.

5. (D) Inguinal lymph nodes also appear hyperechoic and can be mistaken for the femoral nerve in a short axis view. Scanning proximally and distally distinguishes the two structures as a nerve is a continuous structure, whereas a lymph node can only be seen in a discrete location.

6. (B) The femoral nerve is superficial to the iliopsoas muscle and is deep to or covered by the fascia iliaca. Occasionally the nerve can be found between layers of the fascia iliaca. The transversalis fascia contributes to the formation of the inguinal ligament and extends to form the separate vascular fascia of the femoral artery and vein. The fascia lata is superficial to the fascia iliaca.

7. (A) The anterior muscles of the thigh are innervated by the femoral nerve, which includes the sartorius muscle and the quadriceps muscle group. The pectineus and iliopsoas muscles are also innervated by the femoral nerve, with articular branches from the nerve supplying the hip and knee joints as well. The gracilis muscle is innervated by the obturator nerve.

8. (C) A higher frequency transducer (8 to 14 MHz) produces the best image resolution for superficial structures. This is at the expense of a limited depth of penetration. A lower frequency transducer (less than 7 MHz) is therefore required for imaging deeper structures. The femoral nerve is typically visualized at a shallow depth, which obviates the need for a lower frequency transducer. Curvilinear ultrasound probes often generate lower frequency waves and, as a result, produce images with poorer visibility due to the lower resolution.

9. **(A)** Patients with true allergies to local anesthetics can develop severe hemodynamic instability, which makes peripheral nerve blocks in general an absolute contraindication. Clinical judgment is used to determine the feasibility of a femoral nerve block placement, and consequently, all are considered a relative contraindication to block placement. A pre-block scan is recommended in a patient with a femoral artery graft to determine the location of the femoral nerve in relation to the graft and if compromise of the graft would occur with placement of the block. In a patient with a bleeding disorder (acquired, genetic, or medication induced), a hematoma formation may occur with placement of the block, which may increase the risk of ischemic nerve damage. A patient with a pre-existing peripheral neuropathy may have an increased risk of permanent nerve damage following placement of a peripheral nerve block. Careful documentation of the preexisting motor and sensory deficit should occur prior to commencement of the peripheral nerve block.

10. **(D)** The proximal portion of the anterior thigh is innervated by the ilioinguinal and genitofemoral nerves, not the femoral nerve.

11. **(C)** The iliopsoas muscle lies immediately beneath the femoral nerve, with the nerve itself appearing as a hyperechoic structure. Muscle tends to produce an ultrasound image of a mixture of hyperechoic lines within a hypoechoic tissue background. Air artifact is due to a lack of a conductive gel interface between the transducer and skin surface. The result is a large dropout artifact. Shadowing, one of a few potential ultrasound artifacts, appears as a shadow on an image and is due to a loss of ultrasound energy returning to the transducer due to beam attenuation from absorption. Bone, gallstones, and metal tend to produce acoustic shadowing due to high acoustic impedance.

12. **(C)** A field depth of 3 to 4 cm on the ultrasound is ideal for femoral, supraclavicular, and transversus abdominis plane blocks. A field depth less than 2 cm is typically chosen for wrist or ankle blocks, whereas a field depth of 2 to 3 cm or 4 to 7 cm is chosen for brachial plexus blocks or infraclavicular/popliteal blocks respectively.

CHAPTER 10

Obturator Nerve Block

Hari Kalagara

Questions

1. The obturator nerve arises from which of the following?
   A. Anterior primary rami of L2 to L4 nerve roots
   B. Posterior primary rami of L2 to L4 nerve roots
   C. Anterior primary rami of L1 to L5 nerve roots
   D. Anterior primary rami of L2 to L5 nerve roots

2. Which of the following is not a branch of the lumbar plexus?
   A. Femoral nerve
   B. Obturator nerve
   C. Sciatic nerve
   D. Lateral femoral cutaneous nerve

3. The anterior division of the obturator nerve lies between which muscles?
   A. Adductor longus and sartorius
   B. Adductor brevis and adductor magnus
   C. Adductor longus and adductor brevis
   D. Adductor brevis and sartorius

4. The posterior division of the obturator nerve lies between which muscles?
   A. Adductor brevis and adductor magnus
   B. Adductor longus and adductor brevis
   C. Adductor magnus and sartorius
   D. Adductor longus and sartorius

5. The articular branches to the medial hip joint commonly arise from which of the following?
   A. Posterior division of the obturator nerve
   B. Anterior division of the obturator nerve
   C. Lateral femoral cutaneous nerve
   D. Genitofemoral nerve

6. After a successful obturator nerve block, the patient is unable to perform which of the following?
   A. Abduct the thighs
   B. Adduct the thighs
   C. Flex the thighs
   D. Extend the thighs

7. A 65-year-old man complains of medial knee pain following total knee arthroplasty. Which of the following supplemental nerve blocks will help with the medial knee pain?
   A. Ilioinguinal nerve block
   B. Iliohypogastric nerve block
   C. Transversus abdominis plane (TAP) block
   D. Obturator nerve block

8. The articular branches to the medial knee arise from which of the following?
   A. Posterior division of the obturator nerve
   B. Anterior division of the obturator nerve
   C. Genitofemoral nerve
   D. TAP block

9. Which of the following nerve blocks is helpful in preventing the adduction of legs during transurethral resection of the prostate (TURP) procedure?

   A. Femoral nerve block
   B. Sciatic nerve block
   C. Obturator nerve block
   D. TAP block

10. The nerve supplying the adductors of the legs exits the pelvis through which foramen?

   A. Lesser sciatic foramen
   B. Greater sciatic foramen
   C. Obturator foramen
   D. Vertebral foramen

Answers

1. **(A)**   The obturator nerve arises from the anterior primary rami of L2 to L4 nerve roots.

2. **(C)**   The sciatic nerve is a branch of the sacral plexus. The lumbar plexus has six branches: ilioinguinal nerve, iliohypogastric nerve, genitofemoral nerve, femoral nerve, obturator nerve, and lateral femoral cutaneous nerve.

3. **(C)**   The obturator nerve divides into anterior and posterior divisions. The anterior division lies between the adductor longus and the adductor brevis muscles.

4. **(A)**   The posterior division of the obturator nerves lies between the adductor brevis and the adductor magnus muscles.

5. **(B)**   The anterior division provides sensory supply to the medial thigh and supplies the articular branches to the medial hip joint.

6. **(B)**   The obturator nerve supplies the adductors of the legs, and the obturator nerve blockade causes weakness to adduct the thighs.

7. **(D)**   The obturator nerve supplies the articular branches to the medial knee joint. The obturator nerve block along with femoral and sciatic nerve blocks is helpful to attain complete analgesia after total knee arthroplasty.

8. **(A)**   The posterior division of the obturator nerve supplies the articular branches to the medial knee joint.

9. **(C)**   The obturator nerve block is helpful to prevent adductor spasms during the TURP procedure.

10. **(C)**   The adductors of the legs are supplied by the obturator nerve, which exits the pelvis through the obturator foramen.

CHAPTER 11

TAP and Subcostal TAP

Sree Kolli

Questions

1. Regarding the transversus abdominis plane (TAP) block using ultrasound-guided technique, which of the following is true?

   A. Coagulopathy is an absolute contraindication.

   B. Low volume, high concentration of local anesthetic (LA) is used ideally.

   C. Saline can be used to identify and open the TAP fascial plane.

   D. It can be used reliably as the sole mode of analgesia.

2. All the following statements regarding the TAP block in the lumbar triangle of Petit are true EXCEPT:

   A. The triangle is bounded by the external oblique muscle anteriorly.

   B. The iliac crest is a useful bony landmark.

   C. The triangle lies anterior to the midaxillary line.

   D. The technique was first described by Rafi in 2001.

3. The following statements regarding the TAP block are true EXCEPT:

   A. The anterolateral abdominal wall is innervated by T7 to L1.

   B. The nerves lie in the plane between the internal oblique (IO) and the transversus abdominis (TA) muscles.

   C. The aim of the block is to deposit LA in the plane between the IO and TA muscles.

   D. A single injection of 20 cc LA will reliably block all the nerves on one side of the abdomen.

4. All of the following statements regarding the TAP block by landmark technique are true EXCEPT:

   A. This technique relies on feeling two pops.

   B. The loss of resistance (pops) is better appreciated with a blunt needle.

   C. The lumbar triangle of Petit is bounded by the latissimus dorsi and internal oblique muscles.

   D. The triangle is situated between the lower costal margin and iliac crest.

5. Regarding the TAP block using ultrasound guidance, all of the following statements are true EXCEPT:

    A. The needle tip is better seen with the in-plane view.
    B. The spread of the LA should be visualized in the TAP plane.
    C. The TAP plane is best visualized in the midline of the abdomen.
    D. It does not provide visceral analgesia.

6. All of the following are absolute contraindications to the TAP block EXCEPT:

    A. Coagulopathy
    B. Patient refusal
    C. Localized infection at the injection site
    D. Allergy to local anesthetic

7. The following statements are true regarding the subcostal TAP EXCEPT:

    A. It is used to provide analgesia for upper abdominal surgery.
    B. The subcostal TAP plane is between the rectus abdominis and transversus abdominis muscles.
    C. The ultrasound probe is placed obliquely along the subcostal margin near midline.
    D. It can block dermatomes T6 to T12 consistently.

8. Regarding the subcostal TAP block, all of the following are true EXCEPT:

    A. It can be a useful alternative for upper abdominal surgery patients in whom an epidural is contraindicated.
    B. Surgery at the injection site is an absolute contraindication to the block.
    C. Incisions below the umbilicus and surgical drains below the level of the umbilicus are not covered by this block.
    D. It does not cause the sympathetic and motor block when compared to an epidural.

9. Complications of the TAP block include all of the following EXCEPT:

    A. Local anesthetic toxicity
    B. Intraperitoneal/intramuscular injection and failure
    C. Motor blockade
    D. Bowel/hepatic injury

10. Regarding the anterior abdominal wall, which of the following statements is false?

    A. The muscles of the anterolateral abdominal wall are the external oblique, internal oblique, and transversus abdominis muscles.
    B. The nerve supply is from T7 to T12 and L1.
    C. The transversus abdominis muscle is the largest of the three muscles arising from the aponeurosis.
    D. The internal oblique muscle arises from the inguinal ligament and iliac crest and inserts anteriorly into the linea alba.

11. A 27-year-old ulcerative colitis patient, with a prior medical history of chronic abdominal pain, on morphine sustained release (SR) 60 mg Q12, colectomy, pulmonary embolism, on warfarin for anticoagulation bridged with Lovenox, had a reversal of the ileostomy. The safest regional analgesia technique for this patient is:

    A. Unilateral TAP block
    B. Epidural analgesia
    C. Unilateral paravertebral
    D. Bilateral rectus sheath block

12. The site of injection of the local anesthetic in the TAP block is between the:

A. External oblique and internal oblique muscles

B. Internal oblique and transversus abdominis muscles

C. Transversus abdominis muscle and peritoneum

D. External oblique muscle and transversus abdominis muscle

13. The TAP block performed in the Petit triangle may not be an effective analgesic method for which of the following surgeries:

A. Cholecystectomy

B. Appendectomy

C. Cesarean section

D. Ileostomy

14. In comparing a subcostal TAP block with a rectus sheath block, all of the following statements are true EXCEPT:

A. Both need to be performed bilaterally for midline incision.

B. Both are effective means of pain relief for upper abdominal surgeries.

C. The site of injection for a subcostal TAP block is between the rectus and transversus abdominis muscles, whereas a rectus sheath block is between the rectus muscle and anterior rectus sheath.

D. A rectus sheath block can provide analgesia for an incision below the umbilicus, unlike the subcostal TAP block.

15. All of the following statements regarding TAP block are true EXCEPT:

A. Bilateral TAP blocks in the Petit triangle can provide adequate analgesia for incisions below the umbilicus.

B. To achieve adequate analgesia for a large midline laparotomy incision, local anesthetic should be deposited in four locations.

C. A large volume of local anesthetic achieves greater spread and coverage of pain.

D. Catheter placement in the TAP block is difficult and unreliable.

Answers

1. (C) Coagulopathy is a relative contraindication for the TAP block. The TAP block depends on spread of LA in a large plane, and hence, it is a high volume, low concentration block. It is used as an adjunct for anterior abdominal wall incisions/drains. It does not provide adequate analgesia as a sole anesthetic as it does not block the visceral component; also, the spread of LA in the TAP plane depends on the volume and site of injection. Saline can be used to hydrodissect and identify the TAP plane without wasting LA volume when seeking the ideal place to deposit the LA.

2. (C) The lumbar triangle of Petit is situated between the lower costal margin and the iliac crest. It is bound anteriorly by the external oblique muscle and posteriorly by the latissimus dorsi muscle. It was first described by Rafi in 2001.

3. (D) The anterolateral abdominal wall is innervated by the anterior rami of the lower six thoracic nerves (T7 to T12) and the first lumbar nerve (L1). The nerves lie in the fascial plane between the internal oblique and the transversus abdominis muscles. Injection of LA within the TAP can provide unilateral analgesia to the skin, muscles, and parietal peritoneum of the anterior abdominal wall from T7 to L1 depending on the volume and site of injection.

4. (C) The Petit triangle is situated between the lower costal margin and the iliac crest. It is bound anteriorly by the external oblique muscle and posteriorly by the latissimus dorsi muscle. This technique relies on feeling double pops as the needle traverses the external oblique and internal oblique muscles. A blunt needle will make the loss of resistance more appreciable.

5. (C) The transversus abdominis plane can be traced from its insertion to the linea alba (lateral to rectus abdominis) and is best viewed in the lateral part of the abdomen. The TAP block provides analgesia to the abdominal wall but provides no visceral analgesia. It should be used in combination with an oral or intravenous analgesia. Observing the spread of LA is key to ensuring you are in the transversus abdominis plane, and the in-plane technique is ideal to visualize the needle tip and facilitates the identification of the TAP plane.

6. (A) Coagulopathy and surgery at the site of injection are relative contraindications, whereas patient refusal, allergy to LAs infection over the injection site, and already exceeded LA dose are absolute contraindications.

7. (D) The subcostal TAP is used to provide analgesia for upper abdominal surgery. It will provide analgesia for areas of the upper abdomen that are not usually adequately covered by the landmark or posterior TAP approaches. The subcostal TAP plane is between the rectus abdominis and transversus abdominis muscles. The ultrasound transducer should be placed under the costal margin, close to the midline, and the upper portion of the rectus muscle identified. In the midline of the subcostal region, the transversus abdominis muscle can be seen deep to the rectus abdominis muscle, unlike near the umbilicus where it is seen only lateral to the rectus muscle. The subcostal TAP cannot reliably block T12 and L1.

8. (B) The subcostal TAP was described by Hebbard and associates for providing analgesia after upper abdominal surgery. The subcostal TAP is a neurofascial plane between the rectus abdominis and transversus abdominis muscles. The deposition of LA in this plane has shown to block dermatomes T6 to T10 with occasional spread to T12 and definitely sparing L1 dermatome. TAP block does not cause sympathetic block.

9. (C) The TAP block is a relatively safe block to perform, and there have been only few reported complications including failure, LA toxicity, intraperitoneal injection, intramuscular injection, bowel injury, and hepatic injury.

10. (C) The anterolateral abdominal wall is innervated by the anterior rami of the lower six thoracic nerves (T7 to T12) and the first lumbar nerve (L1). The muscles of the anterolateral abdominal wall are the external oblique, internal oblique, and transversus abdominis muscles. The external oblique muscle is the largest of the three muscles. The nerves lie in the fascial plane between the internal oblique and the transversus abdominis muscles.

11. (A) This is a chronic pain patient who will need multimodal analgesia to manage postoperative pain. In view of the previous history of pulmonary embolism and Lovenox administration, epidural and paravertebral may not be the safest modes of analgesia. The rectus sheath block provides analgesia for midline incisions but will not be effective for ileostomy.

12. (B) The TAP plane is the fascial plane between the internal oblique muscle and the transversus abdominis muscle. The order of structures in the abdominal wall is as follows: skin, fat, external oblique, internal oblique, transversus abdominis, and peritoneum.

13. (A) The posterior TAP is an effective means of analgesia for incisions below the umbilicus. Cholecystectomy incisions will not be covered by the posterior TAP but will be covered by the subcostal TAP block.

14. (C) The subcostal TAP and the rectus sheath block have to be performed bilaterally for midline incision and are effective means of pain relief for upper abdominal surgeries. The site of injection for the subcostal TAP block is between the rectus and transversus abdominis muscles, whereas the rectus sheath block is between the rectus muscle and posterior rectus sheath. The rectus sheath block can provide analgesia for midline incision above and below the umbilicus.

15. (D) The posterior TAP blocks will provide analgesia for lower abdominal surgeries. For the large midline laparotomy incision, LA should be deposited bilaterally in the subcostal TAP planes and the Petit triangle. Catheter placement in the TAP plane is relatively easy and has been shown to be an effective means of pain relief.

CHAPTER 12

Quadratus Lumborum Block

Hesham Elsharkawy

Questions

1. Which of the following is the most important advantage of the quadratus lumborum (QL) block compared to the transversus abdominis plane (TAP) block?

   A. Suitable for operations below the umbilicus
   B. Smaller volumes of local anesthetics required
   C. Wider dermatomal coverage (T6 to L1)
   D. Safer in patients on anticoagulant medications
   E. Lower incidence of complications

2. In this image from the lateral abdominal and lumbar paravertebral areas, please identify the following:

   A. The quadratus lumborum muscle

   _____

   B. The psoas major muscle _____

   C. The transversus abdominis muscle

   _____

   D. The spinal nerve _____

   E. The middle thoracolumbar fascia

   _____

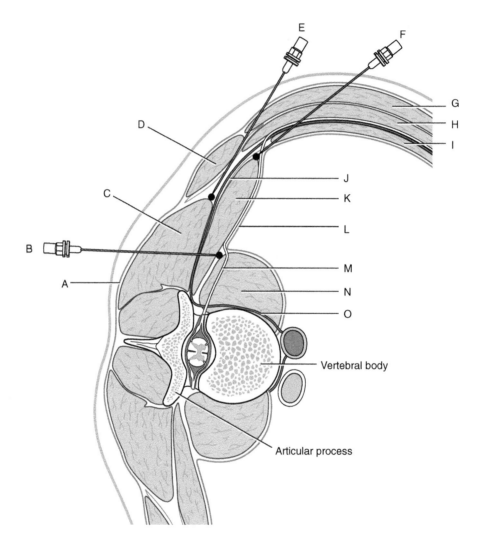

Vertebral body

Articular process

3. In this image obtained during the QL block, please identify the following:

A. QL 1 approach

_____

B. QL 2 approach

_____

C. QL 3 (transmuscular) approach

_____

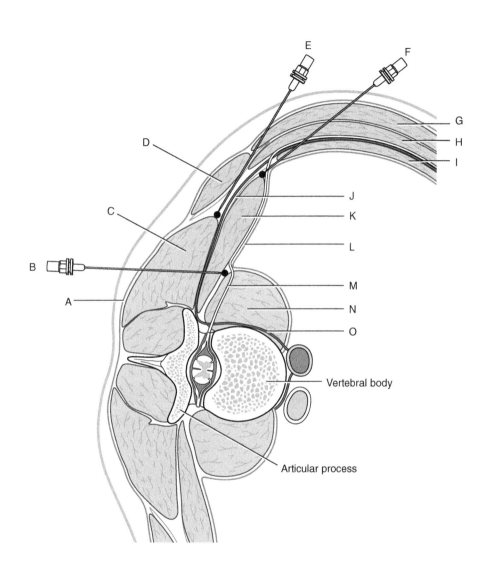

4. Which of the following statements about the QL muscle is MOST likely true?

A. The quadratus lumborum muscle originates from the iliac crest and inserts into the last rib.

B. The muscle of the anterior abdominal wall lies dorsal to the iliopsoas.

C. The quadratus lumborum assists in producing forward flexion of the lumbar spine.

D. The ventral rami pass between the QL and latissimus dorsi muscle.

5. Which type of block is represented in this image?

   A. Lumbar plexus block
   B. TAP block
   C. QL block
   D. Fascia transversalis block
   E. None of the above

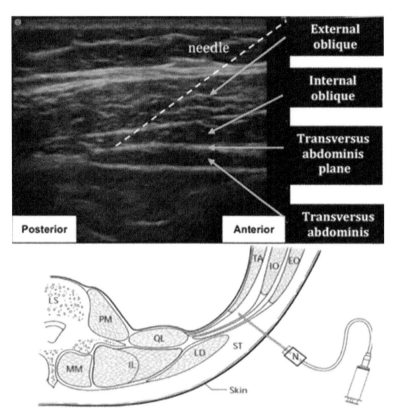

6. All of the following are advantages of QL block compared to transversalis fascia plane (TFP) block EXCEPT:

   A. It offers analgesia laterally over the iliac crest as far as the greater trochanter.
   B. It provides a higher dermatomal coverage (up to T6).
   C. The spread is limited to the subcostal and iliohypogastric nerves.
   D. It covers the visceral component.
   E. None of the above

7. Which of the following is the most important disadvantage of epidural analgesia compared to QL block in abdominal surgeries?

   A. Can preserve bladder and lower limb motor function
   B. Smaller volumes of local anesthetics required
   C. Smaller dermatomal coverage
   D. More sympathectomy and hemodynamic instability
   E. Not safe in patients on anticoagulant medications

8. It is possible to block the central visceral pain conduction with all of the following blocks EXCEPT:

   A. Thoracic paravertebral blockade
   B. Quadratus lumborum block
   C. Opioids administered either orally or intravenously
   D. Epidural analgesia
   E. Rectus sheath block

9. The following statement is true or false: The QL block is safe in patients on anticoagulant medications.

   A. True
   B. False

DIRECTIONS for questions 10 through 13: These items refer to the diagnosis, treatment, or management of a single patient.

   The patient is a 32-year-old male scheduled for a subtotal colectomy. The surgery is scheduled to be performed through a midline incision extending from above the umbilicus to the pubic symphysis. The patient refused an epidural catheter.

10. Which statement about the use of an epidural block for major abdominal surgery is MOST likely true?

    A. It is a complex technique with a failure rate around 20%.
    B. Effective alternatives are available.
    C. It is an invasive technique with the potential for major complications.
    D. Hemodynamic sequelae often are associated with neuraxial sympathectomy.
    E. All of the above

11. Which of the following is the alternative block MOST likely to be offered to this patient?

    A. Rectus sheath block
    B. Bilateral quadratus lumborum catheters
    C. Bilateral subcostal transversus abdominis plane block
    D. Bilateral fascia transversalis block
    E. None of the above

12. The patient developed grand mal seizure 10 minutes after receiving a bilateral QL block. The MOST likely cause is:

    A. Systemic local anesthetic toxicity
    B. Vertebral artery injection
    C. High epidural injection
    D. Total spinal anesthesia

13. One day after the surgery the patient complains of bilateral weakness in the quadriceps muscles. The MOST likely cause is:

    A. Post convulsive manifestations
    B. Possible side effect of QL block
    C. Consequence of kidney puncture
    D. Epidural spread of the medications
    E. None of the above

14. In this ultrasound image from the lumbar paravertebral area, please identify the following:

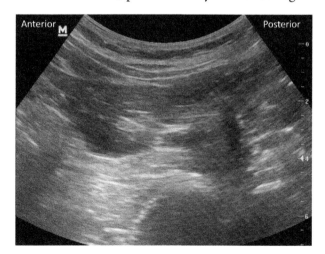

    A. Psoas major muscle
    B. Quadratus lumborum (QL) muscle
    C. Lumbar transverse process (TP)
    D. Local anesthetic (LA)
    E. Lumbar vertebral body

15. In this ultrasound image from the lateral abdominal and lumbar paravertebral areas, please identify the following:

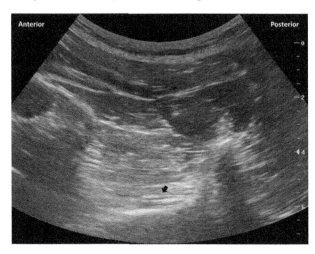

A. Psoas major muscle
B. Quadratus lumborum (QL) muscle
C. External oblique muscle
D. Internal oblique muscle
E. Latissimus dorsi muscle
F. Lumbar plexus

16. Which of the following is the most important explanation for the wider dermatomal coverage of QL block?

A. The QL blocks will block the lateral branches of the thoracoabdominal nerves.
B. There is path between the thoracic and lumbar paravertebral space.
C. The endothoracic fascia is not continuous with the fascia transversalis.
D. The spread distally can reach the subcostal, iliohypogastric, ilioinguinal, genitofemoral, and the lateral femoral cutaneous nerve.

Answers

1. (C) The QL block produces a more extensive, predictable, and posterior spread of local anesthetic, similar to that seen with the landmark TAP block, in that there is subsequent extension into the thoracic paravertebral space. The quadratus lumborum block results in a wider sensory blockade compared to the TAP block (T7 to L1 for QL block vs. T10 to T12 for the TAP block). Ultrasound-guided TAP blocks not are able to produce a sensory level above the umbilicus consistently unless you add a subcostal injection. The ultrasound-guided QL block has been introduced and shown to result in consistent coverage of at least T8 rostrally and L1 caudally. Moreover, the QL block has the potential to provide some visceral analgesia considering its spread to paravertebral and potentially epidural spaces. Potential advantages of the QL over the TAP block are wider dermatomal coverage (T6 to L1), potential coverage of the pelvic and abdominal visceral pain, and longer duration.

2. (A) K

(B) N

(C) I

(D) M

(E) J

The quadratus lumborum muscle is a muscle of the posterior abdominal wall lying deep inside the abdomen and dorsal to the iliopsoas. It originates from the medial half of the iliac crest and inserts into the lower medial border of the last rib (twelfth) and by four small tendons from the apices of the transverse processes of the upper four lumbar vertebrae. The QL muscle assists in producing lateral flexion of the lumbar spine. The ventral rami pass between the QL and its anterior fascia.

The QL muscle tendons attached to the lumbar transverse process under ultrasound usually look like a small boat hooked to a stick (transverse process). The psoas muscle looks like water under the QL muscle and is usually hyperechoic at this level because of its intramuscular fibrous tendon structure and because it is surrounded by thick fibrous thoracolumbar fascia (TLF).

The TLF consists of both aponeurotic as well as fascial connective tissue. Its most important function is providing a retinaculum for paraspinal musculature in the lumbar region. It consists of three layers: anterior, middle, and posterior. Anterior to the middle layer, the quadratus lumborum is situated, which is separated from the psoas by the anterior layer that courses between them. The posterior and middle layers of the TLF fuse laterally to form the lateral raphe, a weave of connective tissue that then joins with two abdominal muscles—the transversus abdominis and the internal oblique. These muscles wrap around to the front, surround the rectus abdominis, and merge at the linea alba.

The four lumbar arteries, one on each side, arise from the posterior surface of the aorta at the level of L1 to L4 vertebrae; they course posterior to the psoas major muscle and are covered by the psoas major muscle and the sympathetic trunk. Between the transverse processes of the vertebrae, each lumbar artery divides into a dorsal and an abdominal branch. The abdominal branches of the lumbar arteries run laterally behind the QL muscle and then forward between the abdominal muscles to supply the abdominal wall. The lowest branch sometimes passes in front of the QL.

The QL blocks the lateral cutaneous branches (LCBs) of the thoracoabdominal nerves (T6 to L1), which arise proximal to the angle of the rib and emerge through the overlying muscles in the midaxillary line to supply the skin of the lateral thorax, the abdomen, the iliac crest, and the upper thigh. The subcostal and iliohypogastric nerves pass deep over the anterior surface of the QL muscle. The QL blocks will block both the anterior and the lateral branches of the thoracoabdominal nerves.

3. (A) F

(B) E

(C) B

This block can be performed via three different approaches with minimal changes in the pattern of injectate spread. **Image,** showing all three approaches with the needles.

After observing the tapering of the abdominal muscle layers under ultrasound, the needle can be directed from anterior to posterior towards the junction of tapered abdominal muscle layers and QL muscle; local anesthetic will then be deposited lateral to the QL muscle and superficial to the fascia transversalis **(QL block type 1).**

By advancing the needle more posteriorly local anesthetic can be deposited posterior to the QL muscle, between the QL muscle and the erector spinae, latissimus dorsi muscle, and serratus posterior inferior muscle **(QL block type 2).**

Alternatively, the needle can be advanced from posterior to anterior through the erector spinae muscle or through the QL **(transmuscular approach, type 3)** described by Børglum and associates to deposit the local anesthetic at the space between the fascial layers of the QL and the psoas major muscles. The same deposition of local anesthetic can also be achieved by directing the needle from anterior to posterior through the QL muscle. The QL 3 may provide an alternative lateral approach to the lumbar plexus block under ultrasound guidance if the needle advanced more inside the psoas muscle and closer to the intervertebral foramen.

4. (A) The QT muscle is a muscle of the posterior abdominal wall lying deep inside the abdomen and dorsal to the iliopsoas. The QT muscle originates from the medial half of the iliac crest and inserts into the lower medial border of the last rib (twelfth), and by four small tendons from the apices of the transverse processes of the upper four lumbar vertebrae. The QL muscle assists in producing lateral flexion of the lumbar spine. The ventral rami pass between the QL and its anterior fascia.

5. (D) See Question 6 explanation.

6. (C) The QL block is different from a transversalis fascia plane (TFP) block. In the TFP, the block needle and medications separate the transversalis fascia from the transversus abdominis muscle. The needle does not penetrate the thoracodorsal fascia, even if the medications spread to the anterior surface of the quadratus muscle. The spread is limited to the subcostal (T12) and iliohypogastric (L1) nerves.

Disadvantages of the fascia transversalis block include a higher risk of peritoneal penetration or liver trauma due to proximity to the peritoneum and absence of any muscles between the needle and the peritoneal cavity; and the block is limited in the anterior abdomen, as only L1, T12, and possibly T11 will be blocked.

Potential advantages of the QL over the fascia transversalis block include higher dermatomal coverage (up to T6); blocks subcostal (T12) and iliohypogastric (L1) nerves and covers the visceral component; and offers analgesia laterally over the iliac crest as far as the greater trochanter.

7. (D)   The QL block can provide unilateral analgesia and can preserve bladder and lower limb motor function. It avoids the sympathectomy and hemodynamic instability following the cardiovascular effects of epidural block. The QL block can be performed in sedated and ventilated patients.

8. (E)   The same as in explanation of Question 1.

9. (B)   The risks of bleeding complications are not known, and there are no specific recommendations. Due to the vascularity of the area, retroperitoneal spread of hematoma, proximity of the transmuscular approach to the paravertebral area and the lumbar plexus, the American Society of Regional Anesthesia guidelines should be implemented in patients on anticoagulants who are receiving the QL block, either single shot or catheter, and risk versus benefits should be carefully considered.

10. (E)

11. (B)

12. (A)

13. (B)   Explanation for 10 through 13:

14.   QL indications: Unfortunately without strong evidence, it is based on case reports and experience. This block shares the same indications as the TAP block, in addition to some surgeries with the incision above the umbilicus, and as a component of multimodal postoperative analgesia for a wide variety of abdominal procedures (any type of operation that requires intraabdominal visceral pain to be covered plus abdominal wall incisions as high as T6). The QL block is conducive to placement of a continuous catheter.

- Large bowel resection, open/laparoscopic appendectomy, and cholecystectomy
- Cesarean section, total abdominal hysterectomy
- Open prostatectomy, renal transplant surgery, nephrectomy, abdominoplasty, and iliac crest bone graft
- Ileostomy
- Exploratory laparotomy and bilateral blocks for midline incisions

Complications of the QL block are related to the lack of anatomical understanding and needle expertise. It is possible to puncture intraabdominal structures like the kidney, liver, and spleen. Extra caution should be taken especially for the right-sided block, as the right kidney is slightly lower than the left kidney and appears smaller when seen with ultrasound.

Transient femoral nerve palsy has been noticed in some patients and attributed to the spread of medication to the lumber plexus and tracking of medication under fascia iliaca. In bilateral blocks with high volume systemic, local anesthetic toxicity should be considered.

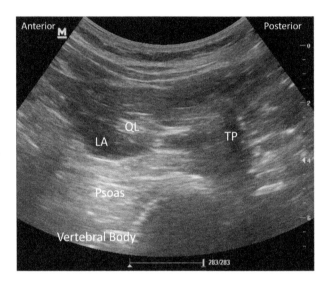

15. Ultrasound images; explanation in Question 2.

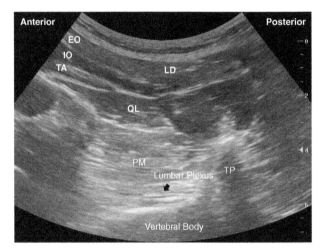

16. (B) There is path between the thoracic and lumbar paravertebral space. The endothoracic fascia is continuous with the fascia transversalis. This continuity occurs dorsal to the diaphragm through the medial and lateral arcuate ligament and the aortic hiatus. The fascia transversalis blends medially with the anterior layer of the QL fascia, anterior layer of the thoracolumbar fascia, and the psoas fascia.

The QL injection and injection anterior to the psoas major muscle can spread cranially through the medial and lateral arcuate ligament to the endothoracic fascia and reach the thoracic paravertebral space posterior to the endothoracic fascia. The spread distally can reach the subcostal, iliohypogastric, ilioinguinal, genitofemoral, and the lateral femoral cutaneous nerve.

This subendothoracic fascial spread from the retroperitoneal space in relation to the QL muscle to the lower thoracic paravertebral space is the base for understanding the major advantages of the QL block versus other truncal blocks.

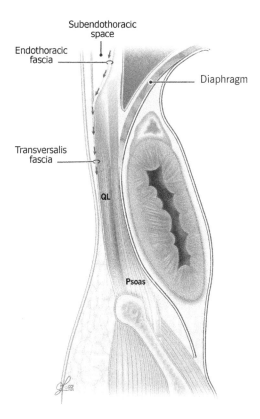

Reprinted with permission, Cleveland Clinic Center for Medical Art & Photography ©2016. All Rights Reserved.

CHAPTER 13

Adductor Canal Block

Kamal Maheshwari

Questions

1. The true statement regarding adductor canal anatomy is:

    A. Anteriorly—sartorius
    B. Posteromedially—adductor longus and adductor magnus
    C. Laterally—vastus medialis
    D. All of the above

2. The adductor canal contains:

    A. The superficial femoral artery
    B. The nerve to vastus medialis
    C. The saphenous nerve
    D. All of the above
    E. A and C

3. The short axis ultrasound image of the adductor canal at the midthigh usually shows the:

    A. Sartorius muscle
    B. Obturator nerve
    C. Anterior division of femoral nerve
    D. Nerve to rectus femoris

4. We have strong evidence to state that the adductor canal block is better for total knee arthroplasty when compared with the femoral nerve block because:

    A. There is less opioid utilization.
    B. It preserves quadriceps muscle strength.
    C. It provides better pain control.
    D. It has fewer opioid-related side effects.

5. The adductor canal block can be useful for analgesia in the following procedures EXCEPT:

    A. Total knee arthroplasty
    B. Tibial plateau fracture surgery
    C. Total ankle arthrodesis
    D. Third metatarsal fracture

6. Identify the sartorius muscle in the following ultrasound image, using a linear probe, through a cross-section of the midthigh.

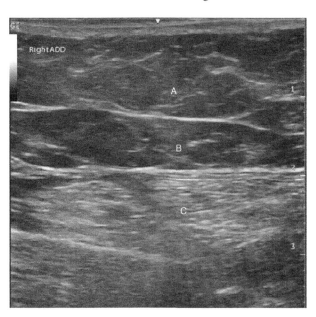

7. In the following ultrasound image, using a linear probe, through a cross-section of the midthigh, the structure in the oval represents the:

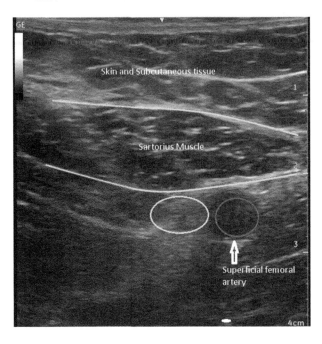

A. Adductor canal
B. Vastus medialis muscle
C. Vastus lateralis muscle
D. Sciatic nerve

8. Which is the true statement regarding the saphenous nerve position with respect to superficial femoral artery?

A. The position of the saphenous nerve is always lateral.
B. The position of the saphenous nerve is always medial.
C. The position of the saphenous nerve is lateral in the adductor canal and medial in the lower third of thigh.
D. The position of the saphenous nerve is medial in the adductor canal and lateral in the lower third of thigh.

Answers

1. (D) The adductor canal is also called subsartorial or Hunter's canal. This is an aponeurotic tunnel in the middle third of the thigh, extending from the apex of the femoral triangle to the opening in the adductor magnus.

2. (D) The adductor canal contains the superficial femoral artery and vein. The saphenous nerve is a terminal branch of the posterior division of femoral nerve. The nerve to the vastus medialis is also a branch of the posterior division of the femoral nerve and supplies the vastus medialis and anteromedial aspect of the knee capsule. Terminal branches of the posterior division of the obturator nerve are also present in the adductor canal.

3. (A) The short axis ultrasound image of the adductor canal at the midthigh usually shows the sartorius muscle and the saphenous nerve (posterior division) as a hyperechoic structure lateral to the artery and anterior to the vein. The vastus medialis muscle lies laterally to the saphenous nerve, whereas the adductor longus and adductor magnus muscles are on its medial side.

4. (B) Evidence is evolving for optimal analgesic technique for the total knee replacement patient. However, preservation of quadriceps muscle strength with adductor canal block has been proven in multiple investigations.

5. (D) The saphenous nerve is the terminal branch of femoral nerve that provides sensory coverage to skin in front of the knee and the medial side of the leg and feet.

6. (C) A and B represent superficial skin and subcutaneous tissue; D represents the vastus medialis muscle.

7. (A)

8. (C) The saphenous nerve is located lateral to the superficial femoral artery in the adductor canal and then crosses over the superficial femoral artery anteriorly just proximal of the lower end of the adductor magnus muscle and runs medially alongside the superficial femoral artery until emerging from the canal with the saphenous branch of the descending genicular artery.

CHAPTER 14

Paravertebral Block

Hesham Elsharkawy

Questions

1. All of the following statements are true regarding the boundaries of paravertebral space (PVS) EXCEPT:

   A. The boundaries of the three-sided wedge—posterior, medial boundary, and anterolateral—extend caudally and cephalad, as the segmental spaces communicate up and down.

   B. The PVS is bounded posteriorly by transverse processes and the rib heads.

   C. The medial boundary is the vertebral body, the intervertebral disks, and the intervertebral foramen at each level.

   D. The anterolateral boundary is the parietal pleura.

   E. Laterally, the space tapers and closes.

2. All of the following are indications of thoracic paravertebral block (TPVB) EXCEPT?

   A. Thoracic surgery

   B. Breast surgery

   C. Cholecystectomy and upper abdominal surgeries

   D. Knee surgery

   E. Renal and ureteric surgery

3. Which statement about the thoracic paravertebral block contraindications is MOST likely true?

   A. Kyphoscoliosis is an absolute contraindication for thoracic paravertebral block.

   B. Thoracic paravertebral block is not contraindicated in patients with severe coagulopathy.

   C. Infection at the site of needle insertion is an absolute contraindication.

   D. Paravertebral and pleural space infections are not contraindications for the block.

4. All of the following are advantages of paravertebral block (PV) block compared to epidural block EXCEPT:

   A. PVB is associated with less urinary retention.

   B. PVB is associated with less Postoperative nausea and vomiting (PONV).

   C. PVB is associated with less hypotension.

   D. PVB had fewer pulmonary complications.

   E. All of the above

5. The following statement is true or false: The spinal nerves in this space are devoid of a fascial sheath, making them susceptible to local anesthetics.

   A. True

   B. False

6. Which statement about the local anesthetic spread in the PVS is MOST likely true?

   A. PVS communicates with spaces above and below.

   B. Fifteen to 20 mL injections cover approximately four dermatomes.

   C. An accumulation of bupivacaine occurs during continuous paravertebral infusion without clinical signs of toxicity.

   D. The addition of 5 mcg/mL epinephrine to ropivacaine significantly delays its systemic absorption.

   E. The absorption of ropivacaine after TPVB is described by rapid and slow absorption phases.

   F. All of the above

7. Which statement about the use of an epidural block for major abdominal surgery is MOST likely true?

   A. Mastectomy with axillary dissection PV injections at T2 and T4 or T1, T3, and T5 is necessary.

   B. Thoracic paravertebral spread is less reliable than lumbar paravertebral spread.

   C. For inguinal herniorrhaphy, blocks at T6 to T8 are needed.

   D. For blocks in the lumbar region, it is recommended that a single injection be performed with small volume.

   E. None of the above

   F. All the above

8. In the classic PVB landmark approach, which of the following is MOST likely true?

   A. Needle insertion is 2.5 to 3 cm lateral to the cephalad edge of the spinous process.

   B. The needle is advanced perpendicular to the skin until the transverse process is contacted.

   C. The needle is advanced 1 to 1.5 cm.

   D. A pop or click may be felt just prior to entry into the PVS.

   E. All of the above

9. Which of the following is not a method for PVS identification?

   A. Pressure measurement

   B. Nerve stimulation

   C. Ultrasound guidance

   D. Loss of resistance

   E. Fluoroscopic guidance

   F. None of the above

10. In this ultrasound image from the thoracic paravertebral region, please identify the following:

    A. Thoracic paravertebral space

    B. Pleura

    C. Paraspinal muscles

    D. Superior costotransverse ligament

    E. Lung

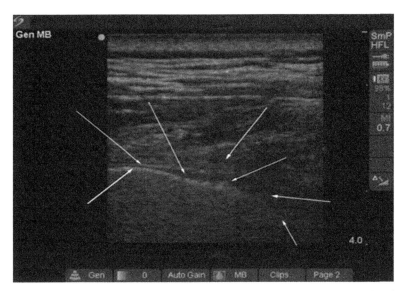

Karmakar MK, Narouze SN, editors. Ultrasound-Guided Thoracic Paravertebral Block. In Atlas of Ultrasound-Guided Procedures in Interventional Pain Management. New York: Springer Science+Business Media; 2011. Available at: DOI 10.1007/978-1-4419-1681-5_9.

11. In this image from a real-time, ultrasound-guided TPVB, which approach was used?

   A. Transverse scan with short-axis needle insertion

   B. Paramedian oblique sagittal scan with in-plane needle insertion

   C. Transverse scan with in-plane needle insertion

   D. The intercostal approach to the TPVS

   E. None of the above

12. Which of the following is the most important ultrasonographic sign for successful PVB?

   A. Widening of the paravertebral space

   B. Anterior displacement of the pleura

   C. Spread of local anesthetic (LA) to the posterior intercostal space

   D. Increased echogenicity of the pleura

   E. All of the above

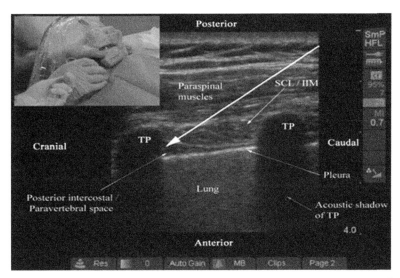

Karmakar MK, Narouze SN, editors. Ultrasound-Guided Thoracic Paravertebral Block. In Atlas of Ultrasound-Guided Procedures in Interventional Pain Management. New York: Springer Science+Business Media; 2011. Available at: DOI 10.1007/978-1-4419-1681-5_9.

13. Which statement about the complications of PVB is MOST likely true?

   A. Failure rate is more than 35%.

   B. Hypotension is never reported.

   C. Bleeding in the paravertebral space is more devastating than a spinal hematoma.

   D. Local anesthetic toxicity is a common complication of paravertebral blocks.

   E. Total spinal anesthesia is rare.

14. In this image from the thoracic paravertebral region, please identify the following:

   A. Thoracic paravertebral space

   B. External intercostal muscle

   C. Internal intercostal membrane

   D. Endothoracic fascia

   E. Ventral ramus

   F. Sympathetic chain

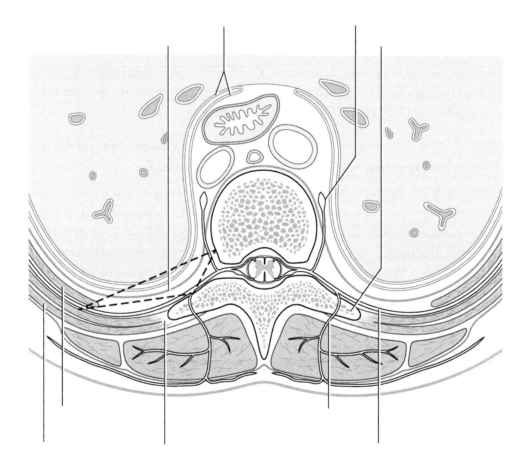

Karmakar MK, Narouze SN, editors. Ultrasound-Guided Thoracic Paravertebral Block. In Atlas of Ultrasound-Guided Procedures in Interventional Pain Management. New York: Springer Science+Business Media; 2011. Available at: DOI 10.1007/978-1-4419-1681-5_9.

Answers

1. (E)   The thoracic paravertebral space (TPVS), when viewed in transverse cross-section is triangular-shaped (dashed triangle in figure below). The base is formed by the posterolateral aspect of the vertebral body/intervertebral disks/intervertebral foramina/articular processes. The anterolateral border is formed by the parietal pleura, and the posterior border is formed by the superior costotransverse ligament. The TPVS contains mainly fatty tissue and is traversed by the intercostal or spinal nerves, intercostal vessels, dorsal rami, rami communicantes, and the sympathetic chain. The spinal nerves do not have a fascial sheath in the TPVS, which explains their susceptibility to local anesthetic blockade. The spinal nerves with their ganglia were found within subendothoracic compartment (SETC), whereas the sympathetic ganglia were consistently located within the extrapleural paravertebral compartment (EPC).

The boundaries of the three-sided wedge—posterior, medial, and anterolateral—extend caudally and cephalad, as the segmental spaces communicate up and down.

The PVS is bounded posteriorly by transverse processes, the rib heads, and the ligaments that travel between the adjacent transverse processes and ribs.

The medial boundary is the vertebral body, the intervertebral disks, and the intervertebral foramen at each level.

The anterolateral boundary is the parietal pleura.

Laterally, the space tapers as it communicates with the intercostal space.

2. (D)   TPVB offers several technical and clinical advantages and is indicated for anesthesia and analgesia when the afferent pain input is predominantly unilateral from the chest and/or abdomen.

Bilateral TPVB has also been used perioperatively during thoracic, major abdominal vascular, and breast surgeries, although in these cases the risks and benefits must be compared to an epidural.

Many different kinds of procedures may benefit from perioperative analgesia provided by PVBs including thoracic surgery, breast surgery, abdominal procedures, and urologic procedures.

In addition to use for perioperative analgesia, PVB has also been used to produce surgical anesthesia. Some centers have had excellent success performing breast procedures under monitored anesthesia care (MAC) and PVB.

Indications:

Thoracic surgery (including video assisted)

Breast surgery

Cholecystectomy, upper abdominal surgeries

Renal and ureteric surgery

Herniorrhaphy, inguinal (T11 to L1 and L2)

Appendectomy

Colostomy/ileostomy closure

Surgical Anesthesia:

Breast surgery, radical mastectomy T1 to T6, axillary dissection T1 to T2

Herniorrhaphy

Chest wound exploration

3. (C) Contraindications to PVB include local infection at the site of needle insertion, paravertebral or pleural space infections, and abnormalities of the paravertebral space like tumors along with relative contraindications of empyema, a tumor occupying the TPVS.

The PVB is performed outside the neuraxis, and the risk for spinal hematoma should be minimal with a paravertebral block. PVB in patients with mild to moderate anticoagulation has been used in several centers. Because of the potential for needles and catheters to enter the epidural space during an attempted PVB and the potential for bleeding into the paravertebral space, this practice is viewed as controversial by many. To date, there have not been any case reports of severe neurologic injury or bleeding from paravertebral block in anticoagulated patients.

Other contraindications include kyphoscoliosis because the chest deformity may predispose to pleural or thecal puncture; patients with previous thoracotomy that may obliterate the PVS by scar tissue and adhesions of lung to the chest wall; severe hypovolemia, especially for bilateral blocks; and untreated sepsis.

4. (E) A metaanalysis of 10 randomized trials to compare the analgesic efficacy and side effects of paravertebral versus epidural blockade for a thoracotomy demonstrated that PVB provided comparable analgesia with epidural blockade after surgery but had a better side effect profile. There was no difference in pain scores between the PVB and epidural groups; however, there was a statistically significant reduction in complications in the PVB group [British Journal of Anaesthesia 2006; 96(4): 418–26].

Single injection produces multidermatomal ipsilateral somatic and sympathetic nerve block as well as maintains hemodynamic stability, reduces opioid requirements, demonstrates a low incidence of complications (compared to an epidural), preserves bladder sensation, and promotes early mobilization.

5. (A) Explanation included in answer to question 6.

6. (F) In pharmacokinetics, a PVB injection of local anesthetics results in ipsilateral somatic and sympathetic nerve block in multiple contiguous thoracic dermatomes.

The spinal nerves in this space are devoid of a fascial sheath, making them susceptible to local anesthetics.

A bolus dose of 20 mL 0.5% bupivacaine injected will result in a maximum concentration of 1.45 mcg/mL in 25 minutes.

Accumulation of bupivacaine occurs during continuous paravertebral infusion without clinical signs of toxicity. This may account for the few reported cases of confusion that resolved after temporary cessation of the infusion.

Ropivacaine does not appear to accumulate in the same linear manner as bupivacaine and can be a safer choice for PVB.

The absorption of ropivacaine after TPVB is described by rapid and slow absorption phases.

The addition of 5 mcg/mL epinephrine to ropivacaine significantly delays its systemic absorption and reduces the peak plasma concentration, but its effect on bupivacaine during continuous infusion is unknown.

Lidocaine, with a shorter elimination half-life and lower cardiotoxicity than bupivacaine, may be an attractive alternative.

Lastly, in cases in which pleural integrity is significantly disrupted, alternative means of postthoracotomy analgesia should be considered as the effectiveness of continuous paravertebral block may be reduced and toxicity may be increased by intrapleural infusion.

7. (A) For a mastectomy with axillary dissection, injections at T2 and T4 or T1, T3, and T5 of 10 to 15 mL each are necessary. The lumbar spread is less reliable than thoracic spread. Individual injections at each level with small volumes are recommended. For inguinal herniorrhaphy, blocks at T12, L1, and L2 are needed.

For single-injection paravertebral blocks that are intended to cover about four levels, a single injection of 10 to 15 mL is placed at or below the middermatomal level of the desired coverage area. With multiinjection techniques, 5 mL injections are used to cover single levels, with 10 to 15 mL used to cover two levels. Returning to our example of a mastectomy with axillary dissection in which the desired covered area is between T1 and T6 (six levels), a two- or three-injection technique is commonly utilized. In the two-injection technique, 10 to 15 mL are injected at T2 and at T4.

For blocks in the lumbar region, it is recommended that individual injections be performed at each level with small volumes (about 5 mL), because spread between adjacent levels is less reliable than in the thoracic region. For example, for inguinal herniorrhaphy individual blocks of 5 mL would be placed at T12, L1, and L2.

8. (E) In the classic landmark based technique, the patient is placed in a sitting position similar to positioning for a thoracic epidural. The spinous processes are marked in the midline, and 2.5 cm lateral to the cephalad edge of the spinous process is marked at the appropriate levels. Infiltration of local anesthesia at the skin entry point is performed prior to advancement of the block needle perpendicular to the skin. The transverse process is usually contacted within 3 to 6 cm. The depth can vary based on the body habitus of the patient and the spinal level. The needle is then walked off the transverse process in a cranial or caudal direction. A cranial direction is preferred because the distance between the superior costotransverse ligament and pleura is longer than when using a caudal angulation; therefore, the margin of safety is greater.

The skin paravertebral distance is greater at higher and at lower thoracic levels.

Body mass index (BMI) significantly influences the distance.

In the T7 to T9 region, the distance is significantly less influenced by the BMI.

9. (F) Multiple techniques have been described to advance a needle and locate the PVS including a landmark technique with loss of resistance to identify the PVS, use of a nerve stimulator to confirm needle proximity to the ventral rami, monitoring injection pressure to identify the PVS, use of ultrasound to guide needles and confirm injection into the PBS, and fluoroscopic needle guidance.

A subtle loss of resistance can be used to identify needle entry into the PVS. This can be felt manually or a loss of resistance syringe can be attached to the needle and loss of resistance to air or saline can be used to identify when the needle tip passes through the superior costotransverse ligament and enters the paravertebral space.

This "give" or loss of resistance is not as definite as in identification of the needle entry into the epidural space. Therefore, it is advised not to advance the needle more than 1 to 2 cm past the transverse process. Reports of unpredictable spread, failure rate, and complications have prompted modifications in the technique to identify the PVS.

Wheeler and associates (2001) described a nerve-stimulation technique to identify the PVS. Using a landmark approach, a stimulating needle set at 2 to 3 mA was advanced toward the transverse process. Contraction of the paraspinous muscles occurs due to direct stimulation by the advancing needle. As the needle tip enters the costotransverse ligament the paraspinous muscle contractions cease. A loss of resistance may also be detected. If the needle is near the PVS, the spinal nerve will be stimulated, and muscular contractions of the intercostal or abdominal muscles are observed or experienced by the patient. These twitches should be in the appropriate dermatomal distribution for the intended block. The stimulating current is lowered until loss of contractions, around 0.5 mA. This indicates the needle is very near the spinal nerve and likely in the PVS. The local anesthetic is then injected.

TPVB is traditionally performed using surface anatomic landmarks. There has been an increase in the use of ultrasound to enhance the safety and efficacy of TPVB. Needle advancement can be monitored in real time either in-plane or out-of-plane with hydro-localization. This may reduce the risk of pneumothorax as well as allow identification of needle entry into the PVS. Observation of the pleura and flow of saline or local anesthetic can provide further confirmation that the needle tip or catheter is in the paravertebral space.

Pressure measurement may be used to verify that the costotransverse ligament is passed. A sudden lowering of pressure is observed followed by "pressure inversion" when the expiratory pressure exceeds the inspiratory pressure.

The acoustic pressure assisted device (APAD) uses pressure monitoring and is successfully used for epidural catheterization but may also be used for paravertebral space location.

10. The image is of a transverse sonogram of the thoracic paravertebral region with the ultrasound beam being insonated between two adjacent transverse processes. Note that the acoustic shadow of the transverse process is now less obvious and parts of the TPVS and the anteromedial reflection of the pleura are now visible. The superior costotransverse ligament (SCL), which forms the posterior border of the TPVS, is also visible, and it blends laterally with the internal intercostal membrane, which forms the posterior border of the posterior intercostal space. The communication between the TPVS and the posterior intercostal space is also clearly seen.

11. (B) Real-time, ultrasound-guided TPVB can be performed using any one of three different approaches:
   a. Transverse scan with short-axis needle insertion
   b. Paramedian oblique sagittal scan with in-plane needle insertion
   c. Transverse scan with in-plane needle insertion or the intercostal approach to the TPVS

12. (E)   Note the widening of the paravertebral space, the anterior displacement of the pleura, and the spread of local anesthetic (LA) to the posterior intercostal space laterally.

In any approach the most important sign is widening of the paravertebral space and anterior displacement of the parietal pleura during the injection and increased echogenicity of the pleura.

13. (E)   Complications include:

Infection: A strict aseptic technique should be used.

Hematoma: Avoid multiple needle insertions in anticoagulated patients.

Local anesthetic toxicity (rare): Large volumes of long-acting anesthetic should be reconsidered in older and frail patients. Consider using chloroprocaine for skin infiltration to decrease the total dose/volume of the more toxic, long-acting local anesthetic.

Nerve injury: Local anesthetic should never be injected when the patient complains of severe pain or exhibits a withdrawal reaction on injection.

Total spinal anesthesia (rare): Avoid medial angulation of the needle, which may result in an inadvertent epidural or subarachnoid needle placement. Aspirate before injection (for blood and CSF).

Epidural spread

Quadriceps muscle weakness: This may occur when the levels are not accurately determined and the levels below L1 are blocked (femoral nerve; L2 to L4).

Paravertebral muscle pain: Resembling a muscle spasm, this is occasionally seen, particularly in young muscular men and when a larger Tuohy needle is used. Injection of local anesthetic into the paravertebral muscle before needle insertion and the use of a smaller gauge (e.g., 22 gauge).

Horner's syndrome: Ipsilateral or bilateral, this syndrome is caused by the spread of anesthetic to stellate ganglion or preganglionic high thoracic fibers.

Failure: 10%

IV placement: 3%

PDPH: 1.5%

Ipsilateral arm sensory changes: Spread to T1 component of brachial plexus

Pulmonary hemorrhage: One report with block following previous thoracic surgery

Pleural puncture: 1%

Pneumothorax: 0.5%

14.   The thoracic paravertebral space (TPVS), when viewed in transverse cross-section, is triangular-shaped (dashed triangle in figure below). The base is formed by the posterolateral aspect of the vertebral body/intervertebral disks/intervertebral foramina/articular processes. The anterolateral border is formed by the parietal pleura, and the posterior border is formed by the **superior costotransverse ligament.** The TPVS contains mainly fatty tissue and is traversed by the intercostal or spinal nerves, intercostal vessels, dorsal rami, rami communicantes, and the sympathetic chain. The spinal nerves do not have a fascial sheath in the TPVS, which explains their susceptibility to local anesthetic blockade. The spinal nerves with their ganglia were found within SETC, whereas the sympathetic ganglia were consistently located within the EPC. The TPVS contains fatty tissue within which lie the intercostal nerve, the dorsal rami, the intercostal vessels, and the sympathetic chain. The TPVS communicates with the contiguous space above and below, the epidural space medially, the intercostal space laterally, the contralateral paravertebral space via the prevertebral and epidural route, and inferiorly (the lower TPVS's) with the retroperitoneal space.

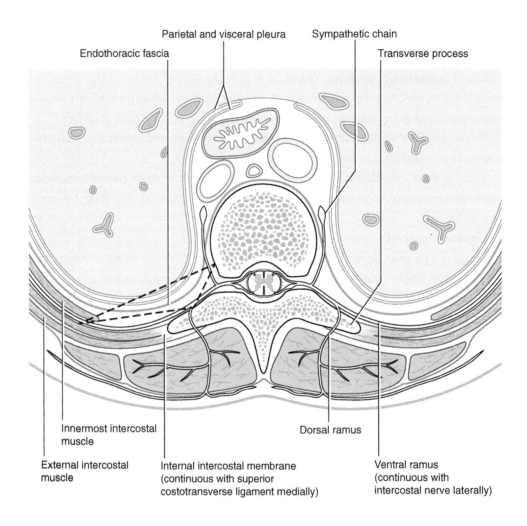

Parietal and visceral pleura   Sympathetic chain

Endothoracic fascia   Transverse process

Innermost intercostal
muscle

Dorsal ramus

External intercostal
muscle

Internal intercostal membrane
(continuous with superior
costotransverse ligament medially)

Ventral ramus
(continuous with
intercostal nerve laterally)

Bibliography

Wheeler, L.J., 2001. Peripheral nerve stimulation end-point for thoracic paravertebral block. Br. J. Anaesth. 86, 598–599.

CHAPTER 15

Lumbar Plexus Block

Hari Kalagara

Questions

1. The lumbar plexus is formed by which nerve roots?

   A. Anterior divisions of L1 to L4 nerve roots
   B. Posterior divisions of L1 to L4 nerve roots
   C. Anterior divisions of L1 to S1 nerve roots
   D. Posterior divisions of L1 to S1 nerve roots

2. All of the following are branches of the lumbar plexus EXCEPT:

   A. Femoral nerve
   B. Sciatic nerve
   C. Genitofemoral nerve
   D. Ilioinguinal nerve

3. The lumbar plexus lies within which muscle?

   A. Erector spinae
   B. Psoas major
   C. Quadratus lumborum
   D. Iliacus

4. Which of the following muscle twitch is used while performing a lumbar plexus block to be a successful block?

   A. Vastus lateralis
   B. Sartorius
   C. Rectus femoris
   D. Quadriceps

5. Which of the following nerve blocks can be used for most effective postoperative analgesia following total hip arthroplasty?

   A. Lumbar plexus block
   B. Transversus abdominis plane (TAP) block
   C. Obturator nerve block
   D. Peroneal nerve block

6. When performing the parasagittal ultrasound-guided lumbar plexus block, the trident sign refers to what space?

   A. Interspinous space
   B. Interlaminar space
   C. Intertransverse space
   D. Interforaminal space

7. Which of the following landmarks are used for the classic Winnie approach for lumbar plexus block?

   A. Greater trochanter, ischial tuberosity, and spinous process
   B. Intercristal line, spinous process, and posterior superior iliac spine
   C. Intercristal line, sacral hiatus, and spinous process
   D. Intercristal line, greater trochanter, and sacral hiatus

8. After performing psoas compartment block, which of the following is the first sign used to assess the success of the blockade?

    A. Loss of sensation in the lateral leg
    B. Loss of sensation in posterior thigh
    C. Loss of sensation in medial leg
    D. Loss of sensation in the foot

9. An 80 kg patient is receiving 40 mg of LMWH enoxaparin (Lovenox) once daily for deep vein thrombosis (DVT) prophylaxis. According to the American Society of Regional Anesthesia (ASRA) guidelines, how much duration is needed from the last dose to perform a lumbar plexus block?

    A. 6 hours
    B. 4 hours
    C. 24 hours
    D. 12 hours

10. After performing a single-shot lumbar plexus block with 30 mL of 0.5% ropivacaine, the patient is unable to move both the lower legs. Which of the following is the most common complication encountered in this patient?

    A. Epidural block
    B. Femoral nerve block
    C. Sciatic nerve block
    D. Obturator nerve block

11. While performing a lumbar plexus block, the patient has hamstring muscle twitches. What is your interpretation regarding needle position, and how would you redirect the needle to perform a successful block?

    A. The needle is too superficial; advance the needle deeper.
    B. The needle is too medial; advance the needle deeper.
    C. The needle is too caudal; withdraw and advance the needle cranially.
    D. The needle is too deep; advance the needle deeper.

12. After performing a lumbar plexus block in a 60 kg patient receiving 120 mg of LMWH enoxaparin (Lovenox) daily, the patient becomes hypotensive, and labs show low hemoglobin. Which of the following complications due to lumbar plexus block may have occurred in this patient?

    A. Epidural block
    B. Spinal block
    C. Nerve injury
    D. Retroperitoneal hematoma

Answers

1. (A) The lumbar plexus arises for the anterior divisions of L1 to L4 nerve roots. It may also receive contributions from T12 nerve root in 50% of cases (Farag and Mounir-Soliman 2017).

2. (B) The lumbar plexus has six branches: ilioinguinal nerve, iliohypogastric nerve, genito-femoral nerve, lateral femoral cutaneous nerve, obturator nerve, and femoral nerve. The sciatic nerve is a branch of the sacral plexus (Farag and Mounir-Soliman 2017).

3. (B) The lumbar plexus lies most commonly within the posterior one-third of the psoas major muscle, anterior to the transverse processes of the lumbar vertebrae (Farag and Mounir-Soliman 2017).

4. (D) The femoral nerve is a branch of the lumbar plexus. Quadriceps twitch from stimulation of the femoral nerve is most commonly taken as an endpoint for a successful lumbar plexus block (Farag and Mounir-Soliman 2017).

5. (A) The lumbar plexus by its six branches covers most of the anterior, medial, and lateral thigh. A lumbar plexus block provides superior analgesia for hip arthroplasty (Farag and Mounir-Soliman 2017).

6. (C) Ultrasound-guided lumbar plexus blocks are gaining popularity and can be done safely. The most important landmark when doing a parasagittal approach is to identify inter-transverse spaces and the psoas major muscle in between these spaces. These intertransverse spaces are known as the trident sign. The lumbar plexus lies with the posterior one-third of the psoas muscle (Farag and Mounir-Soliman 2017).

7. (B) An intercristal line is drawn at L4/L5 and another parallel with the spine through the posterior superior iliac spine (PSIS). The needle is inserted at the intersection of these lines with a slight medial inclination. The needle should be between the transverse processes of L4 and L5 in the landmark Winnie technique (Farag and Mounir-Soliman 2017).

8. (C) By using quadriceps twitch as an endpoint when performing lumbar plexus blocks, loss of sensation on the medial leg supplied by saphenous nerve- branch of femoral nerve is the first sign for a successful block (Farag and Mounir-Soliman 2017).

9. (D) Lumbar plexus block is considered a deep block and ASRA recommends following the same guidelines regarding anticoagulation as neuraxial blocks. A 12-hour period should lapse from the last dose of prophylactic LMWH enoxaparin (Lovenox) to perform lumbar plexus block (Farag and Mounir-Soliman 2017).

10. (A) The lumbar plexus still carry the dural sleeve, and large volumes of local anesthetics injected may cause epidural block. The patient should be observed for hypotension and bilateral block following large volume single injections of local anesthetic solutions into lumbar plexus blocks (Farag and Mounir-Soliman 2017).

11. (C) Twitches of the hamstring muscles indicate stimulation of the sacral plexus. This implies the needle is too caudal, so the needle should be withdrawn and reinserted cranially. Quadriceps twitch is the accepted response for a successful lumbar plexus block (Farag and Mounir-Soliman 2017).

12. (D) The lumbar plexus block is a deep block, and many visceral retroperitoneal organs and blood vessels lie close to the plexus. When the block is performed at a higher level, inadvertent kidney and vascular puncture may happen and cause retroperitoneal hematoma. This block is not safe to perform in patients taking large doses of enoxaparin (Lovenox) (Farag and Mounir-Soliman 2017).

Bibliography

Farag, E., Mounir-Soliman, L. (Eds.), 2017. Brown's Atlas of Regional Anesthesia, fifth ed. Elsevier, Philadelphia.

CHAPTER 16

Popliteal Block

Maria Yared

Questions

1. Which muscle is lateral to the sciatic nerve when it reaches the popliteal fossa?

    A. Semimembranosus muscle
    B. Semitendinosus muscle
    C. Gastrocnemius muscle
    D. Biceps femoris muscle

2. Which of the following will be completely covered by the popliteal block?

    A. Proximal tibia
    B. Distal tibia
    C. Gastrocnemius tendons
    D. First and second toes
    E. B, C, and D
    F. All of the above

3. A patient is scheduled for an Achilles tendon repair and has a history of a femoral-popliteal bypass. On ultrasound, the typical vascular structures you use to orient yourself are not distinct, and it is difficult for you to confirm the location of the sciatic nerve due to scar tissue. You decide to use the nerve stimulator simultaneously with the ultrasound. When using nerve stimulation to identify the proper location for performing the popliteal block, you know you are in the correct location if your stimulation results in:

    A. Plantar flexion
    B. Dorsiflexion
    C. Eversion
    D. Inversion
    E. Paresthesias of the medial lower leg
    F. All of the above
    G. A and D
    H. B and C

4. It is dangerous to inject local anesthetic within the sheath between the posterior tibial nerve and common peroneal nerve.

    A. True
    B. False

5. The common peroneal nerve is larger than the posterior tibial nerve.

    A. True
    B. False

6. As you move the ultrasound probe cephalad, the common peroneal nerve will join the tibial nerve from the patient's lateral side.

   A. True
   B. False

7. What is the dumbbell sign?

   A. An ultrasound artifact
   B. When the biceps femoris, semimembranosus, and semitendinosus tendons are accentuated upon flexion of the knee
   C. The merging of the common peroneal and posterior tibial nerves
   D. When the block achieves sensory blockade without motor blockade

8. What is the seesaw sign?

   A. Nerve stimulation resulting in both plantar flexion and dorsiflexion
   B. The waxing and waning of neurological symptoms in the setting of local anesthetic toxicity
   C. When the foot twitching caused by nerve stimulation resolves after injecting local anesthetic
   D. The common peroneal and posterior tibial nerves moving as a result of plantar flexion and dorsiflexion of the foot

9. When choosing to place a catheter, which location is most ideal in the setting of a below the knee amputation (BKA)?

   A. Femoral nerve catheter
   B. Adductor canal catheter
   C. Subgluteal sciatic catheter
   D. Popliteal sciatic catheter

10. You decide to perform the popliteal fossa block with the patient in the supine position because the patient has an external fixation device at the ankle. You insert your needle and notice that it is a few centimeters inferior to the sciatic nerve. In order to redirect your needle closer to the nerve, you:

    A. Lift your hand upward to direct the needle more inferior and deep
    B. Lift your hand upward to direct the needle more inferior and superficial (toward the interface between the skin and the ultrasound probe)
    C. Move your hand downward to direct the needle more superior and deep
    D. Move your hand downward to direct the needle more superior and superficial

11. From lateral to medial, the order in which anatomic structures are seen is:

    A. Biceps femoris muscle, common peroneal nerve, posterior tibial nerve, popliteal artery, semitendinosus muscle, semimembranosus muscle
    B. Biceps femoris muscle, posterior tibial nerve, common peroneal nerve, popliteal artery, semitendinosus muscle, semimembranosus muscle
    C. Biceps femoris muscle, popliteal artery, common peroneal nerve, posterior tibial nerve, semitendinosus muscle, semimembranosus muscle
    D. Semimembranosus muscle, semitendinosus muscle, common peroneal nerve, posterior tibial nerve, popliteal artery, biceps femoris muscle

12. The surgeon is planning to perform a BKA on a patient without using a tourniquet. This patient has multiple comorbidities, including congestive heart failure, coronary artery disease, stroke, and chronic kidney disease. Therefore you decide to perform a surgical block on the patient in order to avoid general anesthesia. You plan to perform a:

    A. Single-shot popliteal block and adductor canal block using ropivacaine 0.2%
    B. Single-shot popliteal block and adductor canal block using ropivacaine 0.5%
    C. Single-shot subgluteal sciatic nerve block and femoral nerve block using ropivacaine 0.2%
    D. Single-shot subgluteal sciatic nerve block and femoral nerve block using ropivacaine 0.5%

For questions 13 to 15, please refer to the ultrasound image below.

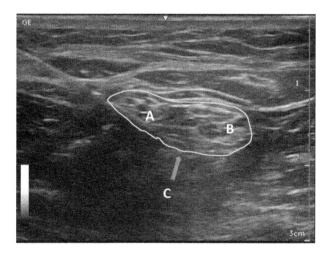

13. Identify letter A:

    A. Popliteal artery
    B. Popliteal vein
    C. Posterior tibial nerve
    D. Common peroneal nerve

14. Identify letter B:

    A. Semitendinosus tendon
    B. Semimembranosus tendon
    C. Posterior tibial nerve
    D. Common peroneal nerve

15. Identify letter C:

    A. Perineurium
    B. Epineurium
    C. Gastrocnemius muscle fascial layer
    D. Fascicles

Answers

1. (D) Semimembranosus and semitendinosus muscles are medial to the nerve. Gastrocnemius muscles are caudad both medially and laterally.

2. (E) The popliteal block anesthetizes S2 to S4 and results in anesthesia of the distal two-thirds of the lower leg. The area between the first toe and second toe is innervated by the deep peroneal nerve; the top of those toes is innervated by the superficial peroneal nerve; and the bottom is innervated by the medial plantar nerve (all from the sciatic distribution). The proximal tibia and tibial plateau are innervated by the femoral nerve and can be covered with an adductor canal block.

3. (G) Do not confuse local muscle twitches for nerve stimulation. Stimulation of the common peroneal nerve leads to eversion and dorsiflexion of the foot. Stimulation of the posterior tibial nerve is recognized by inversion and plantar flexion of the foot and is the preferred response because it is associated with higher block success; this is an adequate location for the block as long as the stimulation is obtained at least 7 cm cephalad from the popliteal crease. If slight movements of the needle lead to changes in motor response from one nerve to the other, it indicates that you are cephalad to where the sciatic nerve branches. Paresthesias of the medial lower leg occur when stimulating the saphenous nerve.

4. (B) The division of the sciatic nerve into the posterior tibial and common peroneal nerves occurs at variable distances from the popliteal crease. Usually, the goal is to block the sciatic nerve 1 to 2 cm before it divides and to inject the local anesthetic around the sciatic nerve or within the epineurium. There may be occasions when you deem it preferable to perform the block at the division or slightly caudad to it. For example, in a morbidly obese patient, moving the ultrasound probe more cephalad can place the nerve very deep, making imaging of the needle and nerve difficult. In this situation, aiming your needle in between the common peroneal and posterior tibial nerves and penetrating their common connective tissue sheath, the epineurium, is acceptable. It is safe to inject within the epineurium, which can cause fascicles to spread apart, but it is not safe to inject within the perineurium. Once within the perineurium, there is injection resistance and injection can cause fascicle volume to increase, which in turn can cause nerve damage.

5. (B) The posterior tibial nerve is larger than the common peroneal nerve.

6. (A) This is one of the reasons why it is important to know the orientation of your ultrasound probe. The classic approach is to have the left side of the screen correlate with the patient's lateral side. Knowing the orientation of the ultrasound image allows you to find the common peroneal nerve more easily as you move the probe cephalad because your eye knows to focus on the left (i.e., lateral) side of the screen in order to watch the common peroneal nerve join the tibial nerve.

7. (C) As the common peroneal and posterior tibial nerves merge, each nerve resembles the weight portion of the dumbbell, and the connective tissue in between the nerves resembles the bar. This sign helps you find the nerves on the ultrasound image. Once the nerves merge and the dumbbell sign disappears, you have reached the sciatic nerve before it divides.

8. (D) Asking the patient to dorsiflex and plantar flex at the ankle will make the nerves rotate or move in relation to their surroundings. Plantar flexion causes the peroneal nerve to become more superficial, whereas dorsiflexion causes the tibial nerve to become more superficial. Having the patient move his/her ankle in this manner can help visualize and identify the nerves.

9. (D) The majority of the lower leg is innervated by the sciatic nerve. Thus placing a popliteal sciatic catheter would cover most of the patient's postoperative incisional and phantom pain. For a surgical block in a BKA, an adductor canal block would have to be done in conjunction with the sciatic block. If the surgery were an above the knee amputation (AKA), then placing a femoral nerve catheter would be preferable. If choosing to place both a femoral and subgluteal sciatic catheter in the setting of an AKA, ensure that the concentration and rate of local anesthetic are appropriate for the patient. Depending on the patient's weight, ropivacaine 0.1% (instead of ropivacaine 0.2%) at 8 mL per hour for each catheter may be necessary.

10. (C) The popliteal block can be done with the patient in the prone, lateral decubitus, or supine position. Whichever approach you decide to use, the ultrasound image will be the same; it is the needle path and orientation that change. When the patient is prone, lifting your hand upward will direct the needle downward, deeper, and inferior to the sciatic nerve. When the patient is supine, lifting your hand upward will direct the needle downward as well, but this will make it more superficial (closer to the interface of the skin and ultrasound probe) and thus further away from the sciatic nerve. When the patient is supine, you attempt to aim your needle so that it is superior to the sciatic nerve on the ultrasound image.

11. (A) Please refer to the text and images in the book chapter to review the anatomy.

12. (B) For a surgical block of the lower leg, both a popliteal block and adductor canal block need to be performed. The saphenous nerve is purely sensory and innervates the skin of the medial portion of the lower leg. If a tourniquet were to be placed on the thigh, then for a surgical block both a subgluteal sciatic and femoral nerve block need to be performed. Ropivacaine 0.2% is a high enough concentration for a sensory block but not a motor block. Ropivacaine 0.5% will provide both a sensory and motor blockade and thus a full surgical block.

13. (D) The left side of the ultrasound image is typically the patient's lateral side. The common peroneal nerve joins the posterior tibial nerve from the lateral aspect of the patient. Also, the common peroneal nerve is smaller than the tibial nerve. Under ultrasound, nerves have a honeycomb appearance. Arteries and veins are full of fluid, and if not thrombosed or calcified, the interior is blood, which appears hypoechoic (black) under ultrasound. The popliteal artery would have been seen deeper and more caudad; it would also pulsate. The popliteal vein is sometimes missed due to being compressed by the pressure applied on the ultrasound probe.

14. (C)   The posterior tibial nerve is medial to the common peroneal nerve and is larger in size. It is the nerve that appears superior to the popliteal artery when placing the ultrasound probe at the popliteal crease. As you move the probe cephalad, the popliteal artery usually courses deeper, often out of view of the ultrasound image. Muscle tendons may be mistaken for nerves. However, as you track the course of the tendon cephalad, it will disappear as it turns into muscle. Nerves will stay constant.

15. (B)   The epineurium surrounds the entire sciatic nerve. Fascicles are a group of axons that together form a nerve. The perineurium surrounds the group of fascicles. The endoneurium surrounds each axon within the fascicle. This image also accurately depicts the dumbbell sign.

CHAPTER 17

Sciatic Nerve Block

Sree Kolli

Questions

1. Which of the following is NOT true regarding the sciatic nerve?

    A. It is derived from the sacral plexus.
    B. It exits the pelvis from the lesser sciatic notch.
    C. It lies deep to the gluteus maximus.
    D. It runs between the greater trochanter and the ischial tuberosity.

2. The sciatic nerve supplies motor fibers to all of the following muscles EXCEPT:

    A. Gracilis muscle
    B. Biceps femoris muscle
    C. Semimembranosus muscle
    D. Semitendinosus muscle

3. During an ultrasound-guided transgluteal sciatic nerve block, all of the following statements are true EXCEPT:

    A. The bony landmarks used are ischial tuberosity and greater trochanter.
    B. The use of a nerve stimulator improves the success rate of the block.
    C. A high-frequency probe is preferred for deeper penetration.
    D. The nerve is most commonly located in the middle of the bony landmarks used.

4. In regards to sciatic nerve block by posterior approach (Labat 1924), all of the following are true EXCEPT:

    A. The patient is placed in Sims' position.
    B. The landmarks used are the greater trochanter and sacral hiatus.
    C. The posterior superior iliac spine and sacral hiatus are the bony landmarks.
    D. The landmarks include the greater trochanter and ischial tuberosity.

5. Which of the following statement is FALSE regarding the sciatic nerve?

    A. It is the largest peripheral nerve in the body.
    B. Combined with saphenous nerve block, the sciatic nerve block provides complete analgesia for foot surgery.
    C. It arises from the nerve roots L4 to S2.
    D. The landmarks used in ultrasound-guided blocks are the greater trochanter and the sacral hiatus.

6. A subgluteal sciatic nerve block was performed for postoperative pain in a 69-year-old patient with severe peripheral vascular disease undergoing a below knee amputation. In the postanesthesia care unit, he complains of pain in the medial side of the stump. This pain is most likely from an unblocked:

    A. Tibial nerve
    B. Saphenous nerve
    C. Sural nerve
    D. Medial plantar nerve

7. Regarding the anterior approach (as described by Beck) for a sciatic nerve block, all of the following are true EXCEPT:

   A. The anterior superior iliac spine and pubic tubercle are landmarks.
   B. The greater trochanter and pubic tubercle are landmarks.
   C. Anesthesia of the posterior aspect of the thigh may be missed.
   D. A needle inserted too laterally can injure the blood vessels.

8. All of the following are true regarding the ultrasound-guided anterior approach to a sciatic nerve block EXCEPT:

   A. The use of a low-frequency probe is preferred.
   B. In patients with coagulopathy, it is preferably avoided.
   C. A slight internal rotation of the thigh helps to give a better view of the anatomy.
   D. It is ideal for patients who cannot be placed laterally.

9. In a sciatic nerve block using an inferior approach (Raj et al. 1975), all of the following are false EXCEPT:

   A. The posterior superior iliac spine and greater trochanter are landmarks.
   B. The greater trochanter and ischial tuberosity are landmarks.
   C. The ischial tuberosity and sacral hiatus are the landmarks.
   D. The intermuscular groove between the adductors and the hamstrings is the entry point.

10. Regarding an ultrasound-guided transgluteal approach to a sciatic nerve block, all of the following statements are true EXCEPT:

    A. It is indicated for surgery on the tibia, ankle, and foot.
    B. The landmarks used are the greater trochanter and the posterior superior iliac spine.
    C. Combined with a lumbar plexus block, anesthesia of the entire lower extremity can be achieved.
    D. In contrast to common belief, it is a relatively easy block to perform with a high success rate.

Answers

1. (B) The sciatic nerve is derived from the sacral plexus, and it exits the pelvis from the greater sciatic foramen. It then runs between the greater trochanter and the ischial tuberosity, emerging from underneath the gluteus maximus muscle.

2. (A) The sciatic nerve supplies motor fibers to the biceps femoris muscle, the semimembranosus muscle, the semitendinosus muscle, the adductor magnus, the hamstring portion of the adductor magnus, and all muscles below the knee. The gracilis muscle is supplied by the obturator nerve.

3. (C) In a transgluteal sciatic nerve block, the sciatic nerve is visualized in the short axis between the two hyperechoic bony prominences of the ischial tuberosity and the greater trochanter of the femur. The sciatic nerve is located immediately deep to the gluteus muscles, superficial to the quadratus femoris muscle. It is seen as an oval or roughly triangular hyperechoic structure, usually found slightly closer to the ischial tuberosity. A high-frequency probe has less depth of penetration but gives better resolution, whereas a low frequency probe has deeper penetration with low resolution.

4. (D) The posterior sciatic nerve block described by Labat involves placing the patient in (Sims') lateral position with hip and leg flexed to 90 degrees. The anatomical landmarks used are the posterior superior iliac spine (PSIS), the greater trochanter (GT), and the sacral hiatus (SH). Draw two lines joining the three bony landmarks. From the midpoint of the PSIS and GT, drop a perpendicular line and mark where it crosses the line joining GT and SH. This is the point of needle insertion for the block.

5. (D) The sciatic nerve is the largest peripheral nerve in the body and is derived from the L4 to S2 nerve roots. In ultrasound-guided high sciatic nerve blocks, the bony landmarks used are the ischial tuberosity and the greater trochanter.

6. (B) The saphenous nerve is the terminal sensory branch of the femoral nerve supplying the medial side of the leg and foot. Combining a sciatic nerve block with a saphenous nerve block will provide complete coverage for surgery below the knee.

7. (D) The landmarks used in an anterior approach to a sciatic nerve block are the anterior superior iliac spine, the pubic tubercle, and the greater trochanter. The posterior cutaneous nerve of the thigh supplies the sensory fibers to the posterior part of the thigh and will not be blocked in the anterior sciatic nerve block. The blood vessels lie medial to the nerve and will be injured if the needle is placed too medially.

8. (C) In an anterior approach to a sciatic nerve block using ultrasound, a low-frequency probe is used for deeper penetration. It is preferably avoided in patients with coagulopathy, as the femoral vessels are at risk of injury. External rotation of the thigh facilitates the block by improving visualization.

9. (A) The landmarks used for Raj's posterior approach to the sciatic nerve block are the greater trochanter (GT) and the ischial tuberosity (IT). Draw a line joining the GT and IT. Mark a point halfway in the groove between the hamstring and the adductor muscles for the needle entry.

10. (B) An ultrasound-guided transgluteal sciatic nerve block is relatively easy to perform with a high success rate. It utilizes the greater trochanter and the ischial tuberosity as the bony landmarks. Combined with a lumbar plexus block, anesthesia for the entire lower extremity can be achieved. Combined with a femoral/saphenous nerve block, anesthesia for the lower limb below the knee can be achieved.

Bibliography

Beck, G.P., 1963. Anterior approach to sciatic nerve block. Anesthesiology 24, 222–224.

Labat, G., 1924. Its technique and clinical applications, Regional Anaesthesia, second ed. Saunders Publishers, Philadelphia, pp. 45–55.

Raj, P.P., Parks, R.I., Watson, T.D., Jenkins, M.T., 1975. A new single-position supine approach to sciatic-femoral nerve block. Anesth. Analg. 54, 489–493.

CHAPTER 18

Atlas Pediatrics Regional Anesthesia

John Seif

Questions

1. In pediatric patients, what are the most sensitive signs of accidental intravascular injection of local anesthetics in caudal blocks?

    A. An increase in the T wave amplitude greater than 25% of baseline; ST segment changes

    B. An increase in the heart rate greater than 10 beats per minute

    C. An increase in the systolic blood pressure greater than 15 mm Hg

    D. Hypotension

2. The anatomical landmarks of the caudal epidural space include:

   A. The anterior superior iliac spine (ASIS), sacral hiatus, and sacral cornua

   B. The posterior superior iliac spine (PSIS), sacral hiatus, sacral cornua, and coccyx

   C. The ASIS, PSIS, and sacral cornua

   D. The sacral hiatus, sacrococcygeal membrane, and greater trochanter of femur

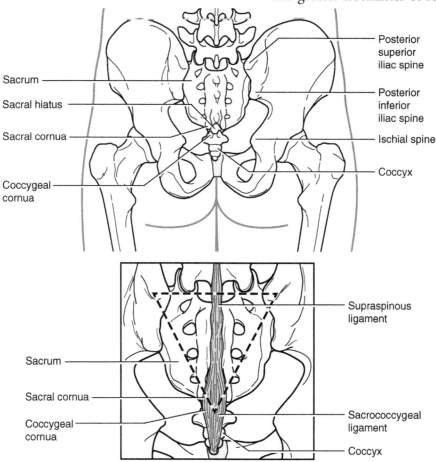

3. What are the anatomical differences between pediatric and adult patients in the caudal and dural sac level?

   A. The spinal cord ends at the L1 level in neonates and at the L3 level in adults.

   B. The dural sac ends at the S1 level in adults and the S3 level in neonates.

   C. The CSF volume/body weight ratio is higher in adults than in pediatric patients.

   D. When performing a spinal block in a pediatric patient, the interspace L1 to L2 is preferred to minimize the risk of spinal cord injury.

4. Why are neonates at higher risk for local anesthetic toxicity?

   A. Neonates have a high level of plasma proteins.

   B. Neonates have an increased activity of cytochrome P450.

   C. Neonates have both a low level of plasma proteins and immature cytochrome P450.

   D. Neonates are not at higher risk for local anesthetic toxicity.

5. How would you manage accidental injection of local anesthetic intravascular that cause hemodynamic (HD) changes?

A. Propofol

B. Midazolam

C. Intralipids

D. Benadryl

6. What fascia is pierced in performing a penile block?

A. Fascia iliaca

B. Fascia lata

C. Buck's fascia

D. No fascia

7. Identify what kind of block is in the following ultrasound picture:

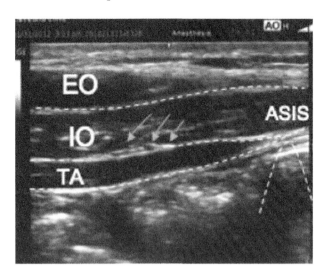

A. Transversus abdominis plane block

B. Rectus sheath block

C. Quadratus lumborum block

D. Ilioinguinal/iliohypogastric block

Answers

1. (A) In 60 seconds, 0.1 mL/kg of a local anesthetic solution that contains 5 mcg/cc of epinephrine will result in an increase in the T wave amplitude greater than 25% and ST changes (the most sensitive); an increase in the systolic blood pressure greater than 15 mm Hg; and an increase in the heart rate greater than 10 beats per minute. The remainder of the dose should be injected over several minutes.

2. (B)

3. (B) The spinal cord terminates in infants at L3 and in adults at L1. But the dural sac terminates in infants at S3 and in adults at S1.

Anatomy	Infants	Adults
Spinal Cord	L3	L1
Dural Sac	S3	S1
CSF/body weight	4–6 mL/kg	2 mL/kg

4. (C) There is a higher risk for local anesthetic toxicity in neonates due to immature liver function which leads to immature cytochrome P450 and a lower level of plasma proteins, which lead to an increase in the free nonionized radical (active form of the local anesthetic).

5. (C) 20% Intralipid 1.5 mL/kg as an initial bolus followed by 0.25 mL/kg/min as an infusion for 30–60 minutes. Bolus could be repeated 1–2 times as persistent asystole.

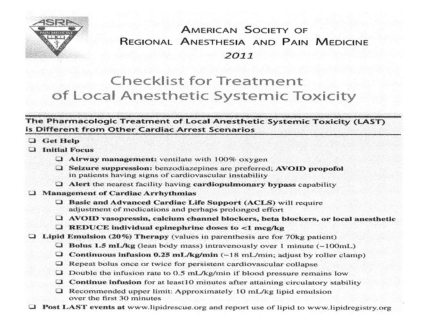

6. **(B)** Using a 25# needle directed to each one of the sides of the shaft of the penis (2 and 10 o'clock positions), Buck's fascia is pierced. Perform a careful aspiration and use 0.1 mL/kg of bupivacaine 0.25% at each injection site.

7. **(D)** The ilioinguinal and hypogastric nerves originate from the nerve roots of the lumbar plexus (L1) and pass between the transversus abdominis muscle and the internal oblique muscle, near the ASIS. This block is indicated for an inguinal herniotomy and orchiopexy procedures. It is especially valuable when the caudal block is contraindicated or difficult to perform.

CHAPTER 19

Neurologic Complications

Suzanne Dupler and Mark Teen

Questions

1. Which of the following is true regarding the incidence of neurologic injury?

   A. The use of ultrasound guidance has decreased the frequency of long-term neurologic symptoms.
   B. Studies show that proximal nerve blocks are riskier than distal nerve blocks.
   C. The incidence of injury after neuraxial blockade is very low and the injuries are rarely permanent.
   D. The incidence of injury after peripheral nerve blockade is common but rarely results in permanent injury.

2. Which of the following is not a risk factor for neuraxial injury?

   A. Epidural technique as compared to subarachnoid technique
   B. Presence of coagulopathy
   C. Concurrent spinal stenosis
   D. Obstetric procedures

3. Which of the following is not a risk factor contributing to perioperative peripheral nerve injury?

   A. Epidural and general anesthetics
   B. Peripheral nerve block
   C. Intrafascicular injection of local anesthetic
   D. Tourniquet

4. Which of the following orthopedic surgeries is correctly paired with the most commonly associated nerve injured?

   A. Shoulder surgery—radial nerve
   B. Elbow surgery—musculocutaneous nerve
   C. Hip surgery—superior gluteal nerve
   D. Knee surgery—common peroneal nerve

5. Which of the following is true in regard to blood pressure control during neuraxial anesthesia?

   A. Local anesthetics, adjuvants, epinephrine, and phenylephrine may adversely affect spinal cord blood flow.
   B. The accepted cerebral lower limit of autoregulation for spinal cord blood flow is a mean arterial pressure (MAP) of 50 mm Hg.
   C. The recommendation is to maintain blood pressure at least within 20% to 30% of baseline MAP during neuraxial anesthesia.
   D. Periods of severe and prolonged hypotension are strongly associated with sustained cerebral or spinal cord ischemia.

6. Which of the following actions is not recommended following an unexpectedly prolonged sensory or motor blockade after neuraxial anesthesia or analgesia?

   A. Reduction or discontinuation of local anesthetic infusion and reexamination
   B. Neuroimaging for compressive lesion or spinal cord ischemia
   C. Corticosteroids if ischemic spinal cord injury
   D. Maintain normal blood pressure or consider inducing high-normal-range blood pressure

7. Which of the following recommendations for transforaminal injection techniques is not true?

   A. The final position of the needle should be confirmed by injecting contrast under fluoroscopy before injecting any medications.
   B. Particulate steroids can be used in cervical transforaminal injections.
   C. A nonparticulate steroid should be used for the initial injection in lumbar transforaminal epidural injections.
   D. A particulate steroid can be considered for lumbar transforaminal injections.

8. Which of the following is true regarding chlorhexidine?

   A. Chlorhexidine solution should be allowed to completely dry on the skin before needle placement.
   B. A retrospective cohort study showed an increased risk of arachnoiditis with the use of chlorhexidine.
   C. Chlorhexidine is inferior to iodine-alcohol as an antiseptic agent.
   D. Chlorhexidine should be placed alongside block trays and instruments.

9. Which of the following is true with regard to performing neuraxial techniques in anesthetized or deeply sedated patients?

   A. Ultrasound guidance has been shown to reduce the risk of neuraxial injury in patients under general anesthesia or deep sedation.
   B. Placing peripheral and neuraxial nerve blocks in an anesthetized adult does not increase injury rate.
   C. Neuraxial techniques should be performed under general anesthesia or deep sedation in pediatric patients.
   D. Paresthesia and pain on injection of local anesthetic are consistent warning signs of needle contact with spinal cord.

10. Which of the following is true with regard to prevention of peripheral nerve injury?

    A. Ultrasound can detect intraneural injection.
    B. Paresthesia during needle advancement or on injection of local anesthetic is highly predictive of peripheral nerve injury.
    C. Data support the use of ultrasound as the superior technique to reduce the likelihood of peripheral nerve injury as compared to peripheral nerve stimulator and injection pressure monitoring.
    D. Ultrasound allows discernment between interfascicular and intrafascicular injections.

11. When performing regional anesthesia on patients with diabetes and diabetic polyneuropathy, which of the following is false?

    A. Ensuring addition of adjuvant epinephrine is important.
    B. Consideration should be given to limiting local anesthetic concentration/dose.
    C. Although current research is still limited, a small number of clinical studies do attest to higher peripheral nerve block success rates in diabetic patients.
    D. Diabetic nerves are less sensitive to electrical stimulation, which theoretically increases risk of intraneural needle placement.

12. What is the incidence of peripheral neuropathy development in patients who receive neurotoxic chemotherapeutic agents?

    A. Less than 25%
    B. 30% to 40%
    C. 50% to 75%
    D. 100%

13. What time period is most closely associated with the diagnosis of postsurgical inflammatory neuropathies?

    A. Within 5 days of surgery
    B. Within 15 days of surgery
    C. Within 30 days of surgery
    D. Within 3 months of surgery

14. Regarding Guillain-Barré syndrome (GBS), which of the following is most true?

    A. Neuraxial techniques are contraindicated in patients with a history of GBS within the past 6 months.
    B. Neuraxial techniques are safe in patients with a history of GBS provided all symptoms have resolved more than one year ago.
    C. There are case reports of reactivation of previously dormant GBS symptoms leading to recommendation to avoid neuraxial techniques in all patients with a history of GBS.
    D. There are too few data to make recommendations on GBS and concurrent regional anesthetic techniques other than to suggest that decisions be made on an individualized basis.

15. Which of the following is true regarding obstetric patients with multiple sclerosis (MS)?

    A. The dose and concentration of local anesthetic are no different than for obstetric patients without MS.
    B. Epidural anesthesia is safer than spinal anesthesia.
    C. Spinal anesthesia is safer than epidural anesthesia.
    D. Neuraxial techniques are best avoided in patients with MS.

16. Which of the following is considered a contraindication to neuraxial techniques?

    A. Complex closed spinal dysraphisms
    B. Spina bifida occulta
    C. Congenital neural tube defects
    D. Previous spinal surgery

17. Which is false regarding isolated spinal bifida occulta?

   A. It is recommended that epidural needle insertion occur either above or below the level of the spinal abnormality.

   B. Incidence in the general population is approximately 10% to 24%.

   C. It is defined as failure of vertebral arch fusion without any protrusion of meninges or spinal cord.

   D. Most cases are asymptomatic.

18. Regarding previous spine surgery, which of the following is false?

   A. Under most circumstances, spinal anesthesia has a higher success rate than epidural techniques.

   B. Neuraxial anesthetics are not contraindicated.

   C. Interventional pain medicine techniques are not contraindicated.

   D. These patients are at a higher risk for developing neurological deficits when undergoing spinal anesthesia; therefore risk versus benefit must be analyzed when deciding between general and regional anesthesia.

19. Regarding diagnosis and treatment of neur-axial complications, which of the following is most true?

   A. A CT is preferred over an MRI.

   B. Seventy-five percent of cases of epidural hematoma will have a fulminant presentation within 24 hours.

   C. Anterior spinal artery syndrome is typically associated with rapid progression to paraplegia or tetraplegia with intact temperature and pain sensation.

   D. A patient who complains of a single paresthesia that is resolving secondary to suspected direct spinal cord trauma from a needle should be followed with serial imaging to ensure improvement.

20. Which of the following is not associated with chronic regional pain syndrome?

   A. Allodynia or hyperalgesia in the territory of a single peripheral nerve

   B. Skin blood flow abnormality

   C. Edema

   D. Hyperhidrosis

Answers

1. (D) The incidence of peripheral nerve injury has remained stable despite the use of ultrasound guidance for peripheral nerve blockade. Studies show that the frequency of permanent neurologic symptoms before and after the introduction of ultrasound is almost identical, about 3 in every 10,000 blocks.

It has been thought that proximal nerve blockades are riskier than distal techniques because of the higher proportion of neural tissues in proximal nerves. There is, however, no compelling evidence to validate or invalidate this despite multiple studies.

Peripheral nerve injuries are common in the first days to a month after a peripheral nerve blockade. They, however, rarely result in permanent injury. On the other hand, the risk of injury after neuraxial blockade is extremely low, but when it does happen, the injuries are often permanent.

2. (D) The risk for neuraxial injury, combining hematoma, infection, and spinal cord injury, is lower in obstetrical procedures. It is, however, higher in orthopedic surgeries, coagulopathy, increased age, and the female sex. The risk of hematoma is also higher with an epidural than with subarachnoid techniques. Concurrent spinal stenosis or preexisting neurologic diseases can worsen injury severity in the presence of hemorrhage or infection.

3. (B) Peripheral nerve blocks (PNB) have not been associated with peripheral nerve injuries (PNI), although epidural and general anesthetics have. The PNB is not associated with PNI even after total knee arthroplasty, total hip arthroplasty, or total shoulder arthroplasty. Peripheral nerve injection injury with local anesthetic is greatest when the injection is intrafascicular in location. This is likely related to the exposure of axons to vastly higher concentrations of local anesthetics compared to with extraneural application, and mechanical damage to the perineurium and associated loss of the protective environment contained within the perineurium. Tourniquet neuropathy can be associated with marked clinical deficits and pathological changes on electromyography.

4. (D) With total knee arthroplasty, the most common injury is to the common peroneal nerve. Shoulder surgeries are most frequently associated with axillary or musculocutaneous nerve injury. Ulnar neuropathy is common after elbow replacement surgeries and persists in up to 10% of patients. The common peroneal nerve of the sciatic nerve is most frequently injured during a total hip arthroplasty.

5. (C) Local anesthetic, adjuvants, and their combinations have variable effects on spinal cord blood flow (SCBF). The reduction of SCBF in the presence of local anesthetics and adjuvants typically mirrors reduction in metabolic demand secondary to spinal cord anesthesia. There is no evidence that either intravenous nor intrathecal epinephrine or phenylephrine adversely affects SCBF.

The previously accepted cerebral lower limit of autoregulation (LLA) was a 50 mm Hg in humans. Many experts now believe the cerebral LLA in unanesthetized adults is 60 to 65 mm Hg. There is, however, a wide variability of LLA among subjects. Preexisting hypertension seems to be a poor predictor of LLA.

The American Society of Regional Anesthesia and Pain Medicine (ASRA) recommends that blood pressures during neuraxial anesthesia should be maintained in normal ranges or at least 20% to 30% of baseline MAP. These recommended parameters, though arbitrary, are inferred based on large population studies that have linked both degree and duration of hypotension to perioperative cerebral, renal, or myocardial injury.

Case reports have attested to an extremely small subset of patients who experience periods of severe or prolonged hypotension sustaining cerebral or spinal ischemia. Although the occurrence of relative perioperative hypotension is common, these rare events stand in stark contrast. It is presumed that because of a physiology reserve that exists between the LLA and blood pressure thresholds below which neurologic injury occurs, the injury does not manifest in most patients.

6. **(C)** Should an unexpected prolonged sensory or motor blockade occur following a neuraxial anesthesia or analgesia, the anesthesiologist must rule out reversible causes in an expedient manner. At the physician's judgment, this may entail reducing or discontinuing local anesthetic infusion and reexamining the patient within an hour. Immediate neuroimaging to exclude a compressive (hematoma or abscess) process should be pursued. If imaging is ordered, an MRI is preferable to a CT, but the diagnosis should not be delayed if only a CT is available. However, if a CT rules out a compressive lesion, a subsequent MRI will be necessary if spinal cord ischemia is suspected.

If imaging rules out an operable mass lesion and spinal cord ischemia is suspected, practitioners should ensure at least normal blood pressure or consider inducing a high-normal-range blood pressure.

The role of corticosteroids in anesthesia-related injuries is unknown. Corticosteroids may have a beneficial effect after direct spinal cord trauma resulting from interventional procedures. However, the use of corticosteroids for ischemic spinal cord injury is not recommended. Corticosteroid-induced hyperglycemia can worsen brain and spinal cord ischemic injury.

7. **(B)** Before injecting any substances while performing transforaminal injection, the final position of the immobile needle should be confirmed by injecting contrast medium under real-time fluoroscopy. Particulate steroids should not be used in cervical transforaminal injections because of the significantly higher risk of neurologic injuries. Although the risk of neurologic injury is much lower when performed at lumbar levels, a nonparticulate steroid (for example, dexamethasone) should be used for the initial injection in lumbar transforaminal epidural injections. Particulate steroids can be considered under some circumstances for lumbar transforaminal injections, for example, after failure of response to treatment with a nonparticulate steroid.

8. **(A)** Arachnoiditis after neuraxial blockade is extremely rare, if it even exists. There are concerns that antiseptic solutions, particularly chlorhexidine/alcohol mixtures cause arachnoiditis. A retrospective cohort study reported no increased risk in neuraxial complications when

chlorhexidine is used as the skin disinfectant. An in vitro study found that chlorhexidine is not more cytotoxic than povidone-iodine at clinically used concentrations. Moreover, if allowed to dry, any residual chlorhexidine carried by the needle from skin to subarachnoid space would be diluted a 145,000 times over. Thus, when used, the chlorhexidine solution should be allowed to completely dry before needle placement (2–3 minutes). Chlorhexidine has been proven to be the superior antiseptic agent, and hence is recommended by the ASRA advisory panel as the skin disinfectant of choice for neuraxial procedures.

To prevent any possibility of archnoiditis by chlorhexidine, the solution should be physically and temporally separated from block trays and instruments. The chlorhexidine solution should be avoided from contaminating the needle or catheter.

9. **(C)** No evidence supports the use of ultrasound guidance of needle placement to reduce the risk of neuraxial injury in patients under deep sedation or general anesthesia. Although patients do report warning signs such as paresthesia or pain on injection signaling proximity of needle to spinal cord, these signs are inconsistent. General anesthesia or deep sedation removes a patient's ability to recognize and report warning signs. A report from the American Society of Anesthesiologists (ASA) Closed Claims study shows an apparent increase in injury rate in patients who underwent cervical interventional pain medicine procedures under anesthesia or deep sedation. The ASRA advisory panel therefore recommends that neuraxial regional anesthesia should not be performed under general anesthesia or deep sedation in adults. Adults with specific conditions such as developmental delay or multiple bone traumas may be appropriate exceptions to this recommendation after considering the risk versus benefit. Conversely, in pediatric patients the benefit of ensuring a cooperative and immobile infant or child likely outweighs the risk of performing neuraxial regional anesthesia during general anesthesia or deep sedation.

10. **(A)** There are no human data to support the superiority of any of the nerve localization technique (i.e., peripheral nerve stimulator, injection pressure monitoring, or ultrasound) over another in reducing the likelihood of peripheral nerve injury (PNI). The use of ultrasound enables the detection of intraneural injection. Current ultrasound technology, however, does not have adequate resolution to discern between an interfascicular and intrafascicular injection. Paresthesia during needle advancement or on injection of local anesthetic is not predictive of PNI.

11. **(A)** Diabetic polyneuropathy is common in long-standing diabetic patients. Consideration should be given to limiting the amount of local anesthetic and avoiding adjuvant epinephrine, as these patients may be more sensitive to local anesthetics. Direct visualization using ultrasound guidance may carry less risk of intraneural needle placement as diabetic nerves are less sensitive to electrical stimulation.

12. **(B)** Approximately 30% to 40% of patients who receive neurotoxic chemotherapeutic agents develop peripheral neuropathy, which may be undiagnosed and/or asymptomatic. Risk of nerve injury is nonetheless increased in these patients.

13. (C) A typical presentation of postsurgical inflammatory neuropathy includes presentation of symptoms in a territory remote from the surgical site within 30 days, but not present immediately. Improvement usually follows, but recovery may or may not be complete.

14. (D) There are many successful case reports involving patients with a history of GBS and successful use of neuraxial anesthesia. However, there are also reports of exaggerated autonomic responses and increased sensitivity to the blockade as well as reactivation of previously dormant symptoms. Currently, there are too few data to make recommendations on GBS and concurrent regional anesthetic techniques other than to suggest that decisions be made on an individualized basis.

15. (B) There are case series that support the general safety of neuraxial anesthesia in parturients with MS. However, in some studies, spinal anesthesia has been associated with postoperative exacerbations whereas epidurals have not. One theory is that demyelination imparts greater susceptibility to the neurotoxic effects of local anesthetics. Epidural anesthesia is therefore considered safer than spinal anesthesia.

16. (A) Previous spinal surgery is not a contraindication to neuraxial anesthesia. Preprocedural imaging to better define relevant anatomy, deformity, and/or surgical implants may be useful. Neuraxial techniques have been shown to be safe and effective in some types of congenital neural tube defects. Anecdotal case reports and small case series suggest neuraxial techniques may be used in isolated spinal bifida occulta. In contrast, there are documented reports of complications arising from neuraxial anesthesia performed in patients with complex spina bifida. Consequently, neuraxial techniques are contraindicated in patients with a history of complex spinal bifida.

17. (A) Isolated spinal bifida occulta is common in the general population, and the majority of cases are undiagnosed as they are most often asymptomatic. It is recommended that epidural needle insertion occur above the level of spinal abnormality, assuming its presence is known.

18. (D) A recent publication reported no evidence that previous spine surgery was associated with increased risk for developing new or progressive neurologic deficits when they underwent spinal anesthesia. Neuraxial and interventional pain techniques are not contraindicated in patients with previous spine surgery. Typically, spinal anesthesia is technically less challenging to perform and is more often successful when compared to epidural anesthesia in these patients.

19. (B) When neuraxial injury is suspected, an MRI is the preferred imaging modality. However, if an MRI is not immediately available, an emergent CT should be performed. Typical symptoms of anterior spinal artery syndrome include back pain at the level of infarction, bilateral radicular pain, and rapid progression to paraplegia or tetraplegia that spares vibration and proprioception (posterior columns). If the only symptom after suspected direct trauma from needles or catheters is a persistent paresthesia that is nonprogressive and improving, imaging is not considered necessary and observation alone may be appropriate.

20. (A)   Chronic regional pain syndrome is characterized by allodynia or hyperalgesia, which is usually limited to the area involved but not in the territory of a single peripheral nerve or dermatome.

Bibliography

Neal, J.M., Barrington, M.J., Brull, R., et al., 2015. The second ASRA practice advisory on neurologic complications associated with regional anesthesia and pain medicine. Executive Summary. Reg. Anesth. Pain Med. 40, 401–430.

CHAPTER 20

Comprehensive Exam

Questions

1. Regarding the transversus abdominis plane (TAP) block using ultrasound-guided technique, all of the following are false EXCEPT:

    A. Coagulopathy is an absolute contraindication.
    B. High concentration and low volume of local anesthetic (LA) is used ideally.
    C. Saline can be used to identify and open the TAP fascial plane.
    D. It can be used reliably as sole mode of analgesia.

2. All of the following statements regarding the TAP block are true EXCEPT:

    A. The anterolateral abdominal wall is innervated by T7 to L1.
    B. The nerves lie in the plane between internal oblique and transversus abdominis muscles.
    C. The aim of the block is to deposit LA in the plane between IO and TA muscles.
    D. A single injection of 20 mL LA will reliably block all the nerves on one side of the abdomen.

3. All of the following statements regarding the TAP block by landmark technique are true EXCEPT:

    A. This technique relies on feeling two pops.
    B. Loss of resistance (pops) is better appreciated with a blunt needle.
    C. The lumbar triangle of Petit is bounded by latissimus dorsi and internal oblique muscles.
    D. The triangle of Petit is situated between the lower costal margin and iliac crest.

4. Regarding the TAP block using ultrasound guidance, all of the following statements are true EXCEPT:

    A. The needle tip is better seen with the in-plane view.
    B. The spread of the LA should be visualized in the TAP plane.
    C. The TAP plane is best visualized in the midline of the abdomen.
    D. The TAP block does not provide visceral analgesia.

5. Regarding the subcostal TAP block, all of the following are true EXCEPT:

   A. It can be a useful alternative for upper abdominal surgery patients in whom epidural is contraindicated.

   B. Surgery at the injection site is an absolute contraindication to the block.

   C. Incisions below the umbilicus and surgical drains below the level of the umbilicus are not covered by this block.

   D. It does not cause the sympathetic and motor block when compared to an epidural.

6. Regarding the anterior abdominal wall, identify the false statement.

   A. The muscles of the anterolateral abdominal wall are external oblique, internal oblique, and transversus abdominis muscles.

   B. The nerve supply is from T7 to T12 and L1.

   C. The transversus abdominis muscle is the largest of the three muscles arising from the aponeurosis.

   D. The internal oblique muscle arises from the inguinal ligament and the iliac crest and inserts anteriorly into the linea alba.

7. A 27-year-old ulcerative colitis patient with PMH of chronic abdominal pain on morphine SR 60 mg Q12, colectomy, PE on warfarin for anticoagulation bridged with Lovenox, had a reversal of an ileostomy. The safest regional analgesia technique for this patient is:

   A. Unilateral TAP block
   B. Epidural analgesia
   C. Unilateral paravertebral
   D. Bilateral rectus sheath block

8. The site of injection of local anesthetic in the TAP block is between the:

   A. External oblique and internal oblique muscles

   B. Internal oblique and transversus abdominis muscles

   C. Transversus abdominis muscle and the peritoneum

   D. External oblique muscle and the transversus abdominis muscle

9. All of the following statements regarding the TAP block are true EXCEPT:

   A. Bilateral TAP blocks in Petit's triangle can provide adequate analgesia for incisions below the umbilicus.

   B. To achieve adequate analgesia for a large midline laparotomy incision, local anesthetic should be deposited in four locations.

   C. A large volume of local anesthetic achieves greater spread and coverage of pain.

   D. Catheter placement in the TAP plane is difficult and unreliable.

10. Which of the following local anesthetics are metabolized by a pseudocholinesterase?

    A. Lidocaine
    B. Mepivacaine
    C. Procaine
    D. Prilocaine

11. According to the manufacturer of DepoBupivacaine (Exparel), which of the following statements regarding drug administration is incorrect?

    A. The maximum dosage should not exceed 266 mg (one 20 mL vial).

    B. Exparel can be mixed with other local anesthetics prior to injection.

    C. Vials of Exparel should be inverted to resuspend the particles immediately prior to withdrawal from the vial.

    D. Exparel should be used within 4 hours of preparation in a syringe.

12. Regarding toxicity diagnosis, an early sign of local anesthetic toxicity is:

    A. Lightheadedness and dizziness
    B. Muscle twitching and convulsions
    C. Cardiovascular depression and collapse
    D. Respiratory depression and arrest
    E. Hypotension

13. According to American Society of Regional Anesthesia and Pain Medicine treatment of local anesthetic toxicity includes:

    A. Epinephrine doses less than 1 mcg/kg
    B. Lipid emulsion (20%) bolus 1.5 mL/kg (lean body mass) intravenously, followed by continuous infusion 0.25 mL/kg/min
    C. Repeat bolus once or twice for persistent cardiovascular collapse
    D. Decrease the infusion rate to 0.1 mL/kg/min if blood pressure remains low
    E. All of the above

14. Which if the following statements is true about local anesthetic cardiac toxicity?

    A. Bupivacaine is the most cardiotoxic drug.
    B. Lipid solubility and high protein binding of bupivacaine are some of the factors responsible for higher cardiotoxicity.
    C. The R(+) isomer very avidly binds to cardiac sodium channels.
    D. Bupivacaine does not release from the binding site easily.
    E. All of the above

15. Amide local anesthetics (LAs) are metabolized in the liver by cytochrome P450 enzymes. These enzymes reach adult activity level by:

    A. 9 months to 1 year
    B. 20 to 24 months
    C. 36 months
    D. 48 months

16. Neonates and infants are more sensitive than adults to amide LA-induced cardiotoxicity due to their:

    A. Relatively larger volume of distribution (VD) of amide LAs compared to adults
    B. Higher baseline heart rates
    C. Lower clearance
    D. Lower protein binding

17. Neonates require larger doses of LAs for spinal anesthesia, and the duration of the spinal block is shorter compared to adults due to:

    A. Larger total volume of CSF
    B. More rapid turnover of CSF than for adults
    C. A and B
    D. Higher glucose content of CSF

18. Chloroprocaine is increasingly used to provide continuous epidural infusion for postoperative pain control in neonates instead of amide LAs because:

    A. It is rapidly metabolized by cholinesterases.
    B. It is rapidly metabolized by the liver.
    C. It is rapidly eliminated by the kidney.
    D. It is has higher binding to albumin.

19. You are asked to perform an interscalene block for shoulder surgery on an otherwise healthy 55-year-old male. In order to successfully perform the block, what landmarks would you use to identify the posterior triangle?

    A. Posterior border of the sternocleidomastoid and trapezius muscles at the level C6 and C7 vertebrae
    B. Medial border of the sternocleidomastoid and trapezius muscles and the level of C5 and C6 vertebrae
    C. Medial border of the anterior scalene and anterior border of the sternocleidomastoid muscle at the level of C6 and C7 cervical vertebrae
    D. Posterior border of the sternocleidomastoid muscle at the level of C5 and C6 vertebrae
    E. None of the above

20. You are utilizing ultrasound to perform an interscalene block on an elderly female who is about to undergo a right total shoulder arthroplasty. How would you identify the dorsal scapular and long thoracic nerves while scanning for the brachial plexus under ultrasound at the proper level?

    A. 2 cm anterior to the brachial plexus located in the anterior scalene
    B. 1 cm anterior to the brachial plexus located in the middle scalene
    C. 2 cm posterior to the brachial plexus located in the anterior scalene
    D. Less than 1 cm posterior to the brachial plexus located in the middle scalene
    E. Less than 1 cm anterior to the brachial plexus located in the anterior scalene

21. A few days after a needle insertion into the middle scalene muscle for an interscalene block, your patient presents with a right side ache along the medial border of the scapula along with a physical exam remarkable for the right scapulae being farther from midline when compared to the left. What nerve has most likely been injured?

    A. Dorsal scapular
    B. Long thoracic
    C. Supraclavicular
    D. Intercostal
    E. Axillary nerve

22. What could an injury to the long thoracic nerve while performing an interscalene block present as?

    A. Chronic pain of the shoulder and weakness of the serratus posterior muscle
    B. Chronic back pain and weakness of the trapezius muscle
    C. Chronic pain of the shoulder and weakness of the serratus anterior muscle
    D. Chronic back pain and weakness of the serratus anterior muscle
    E. None of the above

23. The most common complication associated with an interscalene nerve block is:

    A. Vertebral artery injection
    B. Recurrent laryngeal nerve paralysis
    C. Phrenic nerve paralysis
    D. Internal carotid artery injection
    E. Pneumothorax

24. A 74-year-old patient had a recent fall and fractured her right proximal humerus. She is scheduled for an open reduction internal fixation and regional anesthesia was requested by the surgeon. A peripheral nerve block was chosen to anesthetize the brachial plexus using the supraclavicular approach. In relation to the supraclavicular artery, where will the trunks and divisions lie while using ultrasound?

A. Anterior and lateral

B. Superior and lateral

C. Superior and medial

D. Superior and posterior

E. Anterior and medial

25. A brachial plexus block is performed using the supraclavicular approach for shoulder surgery. A catheter will be placed for postoperative analgesia. For the most optimal analgesia in the patient, the catheter should be placed:

A. Anterior to the subclavian artery

B. Posterior to the subclavian artery

C. Superior to the subclavian artery

D. As close as possible to the first rib

E. Under the first rib

26. After receiving a brachial plexus block with the supraclavicular approach, the patient undergoes shoulder arthroscopy, but although experiencing numbness and weakness in the lower arm and hand, the patient develops severe shoulder pain. Which nerve was most likely affected, causing this pain?

A. Suprascapular nerve

B. Subscapular nerve

C. Radial nerve

D. Intercostobrachial nerve

E. Infrascapular nerve

27. What is the most common complication associated with a brachial plexus block using the supraclavicular approach?

A. Intravascular injection into the subclavian artery

B. Intravascular injection into the vertebral artery

C. Pneumothorax

D. Failed block

E. Phrenic nerve paralysis

28. Which section of the brachial plexus is anesthetized when performing a supraclavicular block?

A. Roots and trunks

B. Trunks and division

C. Division and cords

D. Cords

E. Branches

29. After successfully performing a preoperative supraclavicular block for creation of an AV fistula, the anterior chest wall is scanned using ultrasound. When trying to rule out pneumothorax, what ultrasound sign should be present?

A. Sliding sign

B. Scaling sign

C. Rolling sign

D. Intrapleural air sign

E. Friction rub

30. Which portion of the upper extremity may not be completely anesthetized after performing a supraclavicular block?

A. Lateral portion of the hand

B. Elbow

C. Medial portion of the hand

D. Posterior medial portion of the forearm

E. Anterior lateral portion of the arm

31. A 38-year-old male presents to the operating room for ulnar nerve anterior transposition due to cubital tunnel syndrome not relieved by medial management. The surgeon requests regional anesthesia prior to starting the case. A brachial plexus block using the supraclavicular approach was performed with 30 cc of 0.75% bupivacaine prior to being transported to the operating room. Which one of these signs and/or symptoms is the first to present in local anesthetic toxicity?

    A. Seizure
    B. Lightheadedness
    C. Visual disturbances
    D. Hemodynamic collapse
    E. Shivering

32. An axillary block can be used in all of these surgeries to control pain EXCEPT:

    A. Elbow surgeries
    B. Hand surgeries
    C. Wrist surgeries
    E. Shoulder surgeries
    E. Forearm surgeries

33. Which nerve provides motor branches to the flexors of the hand and wrist?

    A. Median nerve
    B. Ulnar nerve
    C. Radial nerve
    D. Musculocutaneous nerve
    E. Intercostobrachial nerve

34. Complications of the axillary block include:

    A. Nerve injury
    B. Vascular puncture
    C. Hematoma
    D. Local anesthetic toxicity
    E. All of the above

35. Under ultrasound the musculocutaneous nerve appears as a:

    A. Hypoechoic circular nerve
    B. Hypoechoic flattened oval with a bright hyperechoic rim
    C. Hyperechoic flattened oval nerve with a hypoechoic rim
    D. None of the above

Questions 36 through 39: Please match the structure below with the letter that corresponds to it in the ultrasound image.

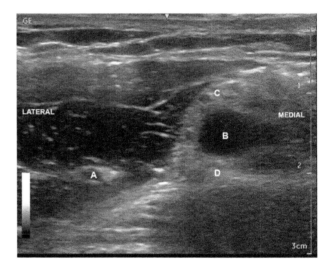

36. Musculocutaneous nerve _____

37. Axillary artery_____

38. Median nerve_____

39. Radial nerve_____

40. An infraclavicular block is typically performed at which level of the brachial plexus?

    A. Terminal nerves
    B. Cords
    C. Roots
    D. Divisions

41. Identify the starred structure in the ultrasound image. Cephalad is to the left.

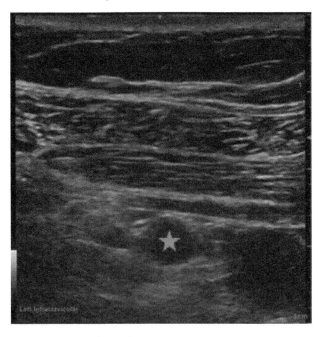

- **A.** Lateral cord
- **B.** Axillary vein
- **C.** Axillary artery
- **D.** Brachial artery

42. Identify the fascial plane indicated in the ultrasound image. Cephalad is to the left.

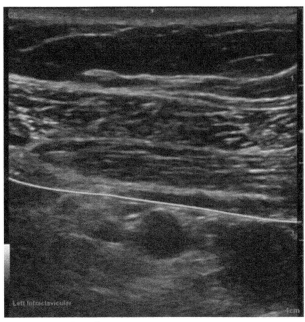

- **A.** Deltoid
- **B.** Pectoralis minor
- **C.** Endothoracic
- **D.** Fascia lata

43. A patient receives an infraclavicular block for radial fracture fixation. Complete anesthesia of the hand and forearm is noted. Upon inflation of the surgical tourniquet, the patient complains of pain under the axilla. Which nerve was not blocked?

- **A.** Musculocutaneous
- **B.** Radial
- **C.** Medial brachial cutaneous
- **D.** Intercostobrachial

44. Identify the numbered structures in order (1 to 3) in the image. Cephalad is to the left.

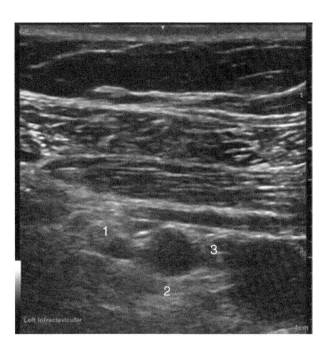

- **A.** Medial cord, lateral cord, posterior cord
- **B.** Median nerve, radial nerve, ulnar nerve
- **C.** Lateral cord, medial cord, posterior cord
- **D.** Lateral cord, posterior cord, medial cord

45. While determining the location for needle insertion for an infraclavicular block, the anesthesiologist is unable to visualize the axillary vessels or brachial plexus just medial to the coracoid process. The best course of action is:

    A. Abduct the arm and flex the elbow.
    B. Scan medially until the plexus is visible.
    C. Abandon the procedure because it is not possible in this patient.
    D. Use a nerve stimulator because the structures are too deep to image using ultrasound in this patient.

46. In a typical transverse scan of the inguinal region, the femoral nerve is immediately deep to the following structure:

    A. The fascia of the iliopsoas muscle
    B. The fascia iliaca
    C. The fascia lata
    D. The femoral artery

47. The base of the femoral triangle is formed by all of these muscles EXCEPT:

    A. The sartorius muscle
    B. The iliopsoas muscle
    C. The pectineus muscle
    D. The adductor longus muscle

48. All of the following are reliable responses of ensuring success of a femoral nerve block EXCEPT:

    A. A quadriceps muscle twitch
    B. Stimulation of the femoral nerve at 0.4 mA
    C. A sartorius muscle twitch
    D. A patella twitch

49. All of the following can be used to distinguish the femoral nerve from an inguinal lymph node EXCEPT:

    A. Scanning proximally
    B. Scanning distally
    C. Scanning in the long axis view
    D. Noting a hyperechoic structure

50. Which of the following represents the MOST ideal ultrasound transducer for performing a femoral nerve block in a 70 kg patient with a normal body mass index?

    A. A curvilinear probe at 2 MHz
    B. A linear probe at 5 MHz
    C. A linear probe at 12 MHz
    D. A curvilinear probe at 5 MHz

51. Which of the following corresponds to the structure denoted by the arrowheads in the following image?

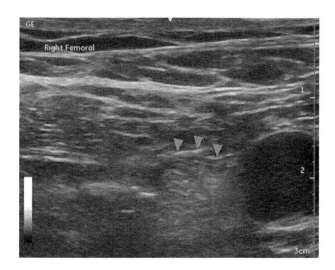

    A. Transversalis fascia
    B. Fascia iliaca
    C. Sartorius muscle fascia
    D. Fascia lata

52. The obturator nerve arises from which of the following?

    A. Anterior primary rami of L2 to L4 nerve roots
    B. Posterior primary rami of L2 to L4 nerve roots
    C. Anterior primary rami of L1 to L5 nerve roots
    D. Anterior primary rami of L2 to L5 nerve roots

53. The anterior division of the obturator nerve lies between which muscles?

    A. Adductor longus and sartorius
    B. Adductor brevis and adductor magnus
    C. Adductor longus and adductor brevis
    D. Adductor brevis and sartorius

54. The articular branches to the medial hip joint commonly arise from which of the following?

    A. Posterior division of the obturator nerve
    B. Anterior division of the obturator nerve
    C. Lateral femoral cutaneous nerve
    D. Genitofemoral nerve

55. The articular branches to the medial knee arise from which of the following?

    A. Posterior division of the obturator nerve
    B. Anterior division of the obturator nerve
    C. Genitofemoral nerve
    D. TAP block

56. The nerve supplying the adductors of the legs exits the pelvis through which foramen?

    A. Lesser sciatic foramen
    B. Greater sciatic foramen
    C. Obturator foramen
    D. Vertebral foramen

57. Which of the following is the most important advantage of quadratus lumborum (QL) block compared to the transversus abdominis plane (TAP) block?

    A. Suitable for operations below the umbilicus
    B. Smaller volumes of local anesthetics required
    C. Wider dermatomal coverage (T6 to L1)
    D. Safer in patients on anticoagulant medications
    E. Lower incidence of complications

58. In this image from the lateral abdominal and lumbar paravertebral areas, please identify the following:

    A. The quadratus lumborum muscle
    _____

    B. The psoas major muscle
    _____

    C. The transversus abdominis muscle
    _____

    D. The spinal nerve _____
    E. The middle thoracolumbar fascia
    _____

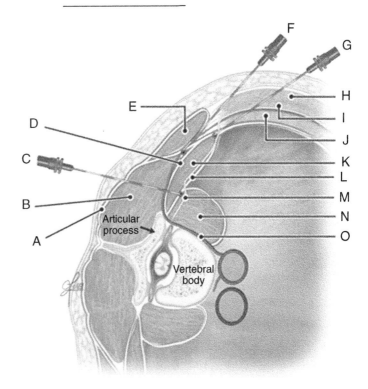

59. Which statement about the QL muscle is MOST likely true?

    A. The quadratus lumborum muscle originates from the iliac crest and inserts into the last rib.
    B. The muscle of the anterior abdominal wall lies dorsal to the iliopsoas.
    C. The quadratus lumborum assists in producing forward flexion of the lumbar spine.
    D. The ventral rami pass between the QL and latissimus dorsi muscles.

60. Which of the following is the most important disadvantage of epidural analgesia compared to quadratus lumborum (QL) block in abdominal surgeries?

    A. Can preserve bladder and lower limb motor function
    B. Smaller volumes of local anesthetics required
    C. Smaller dermatomal coverage
    D. More sympathectomy and hemodynamic instability
    E. Not safe in patients on anticoagulant medications

61. It is possible to block the central visceral pain conduction with all of the following blocks EXCEPT:

    A. Thoracic paravertebral blockade
    B. Quadratus lumborum block
    C. Opioids administered either orally or intravenously
    D. Epidural analgesia
    E. Rectus sheath block

    Directions for questions 62 through 65: These items refer to the diagnosis, treatment, or management of a single patient.

62. The patient is a 32-year-old male scheduled for a subtotal colectomy. The surgery is scheduled to be performed through a midline incision extending from above the umbilicus to the pubic symphysis. The patient refused an epidural catheter. Which statement about the use of an epidural block for major abdominal surgery is MOST likely true?

    A. It is a complex technique with a failure rate around 20%.
    B. Effective alternatives are available.
    C. It is an invasive technique with the potential for major complications.
    D. Hemodynamic sequelae are often associated with neuraxial sympathectomy.
    E. All of the above

63. Which of the following is MOST likely the alternative block offered to this patient?

    A. Rectus sheath block
    B. Bilateral quadratus lumborum catheters
    C. Bilateral subcostal transversus abdominis plane block
    D. Bilateral fascia transversalis block
    E. None of the above

64. The patient developed grand mal seizure 10 minutes after receiving bilateral QL block. The MOST likely cause is:

    A. Systemic local anesthetic toxicity
    B. Vertebral artery injection
    C. High epidural injection
    D. Total spinal anesthesia

65. One day after the surgery the patient complains of bilateral weakness in the quadriceps muscles. The MOST likely cause is:

    A. Post convulsive manifestations
    B. Possible side effect of QL block
    C. Consequence of kidney puncture
    D. Epidural spread of the medications
    E. None of the above

66. The true statement regarding adductor canal anatomy is:

    A. Anteriorly—sartorius
    B. Posteromedially—adductor longus and adductor magnus
    C. Laterally—vastus medialis
    D. All of the above

67. The short axis ultrasound image of the adductor canal at the midthigh usually shows the:

    A. Sartorius muscle
    B. Obturator nerve
    C. Anterior division of femoral nerve
    D. Nerve to rectus femoris

68. The adductor canal block can be useful for analgesia in the following procedures EXCEPT:

    A. Total knee arthroplasty
    B. Tibial plateau fracture surgery
    C. Total ankle arthrodesis
    D. Third metatarsal fracture

69. Identify the sartorius muscle in the following ultrasound image, using a linear probe, through a cross-section of the midthigh.

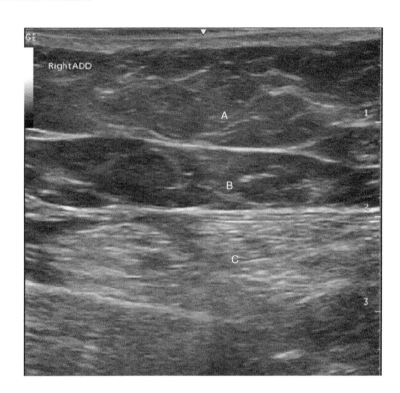

70 In the following ultrasound image, using a linear probe, through a cross-section of the midthigh the structure in the oval represents the:

    A. Adductor canal
    B. Vastus medialis muscle
    C. Vastus lateralis muscle
    D. Sciatic nerve

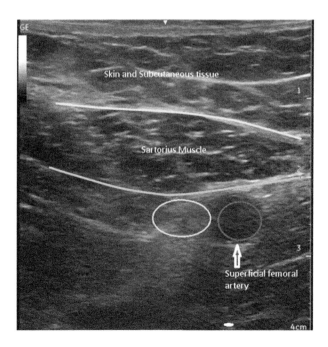

71. Which is the true statement regarding the saphenous nerve position with respect to the superficial femoral artery?

   A. The position of the saphenous nerve is always lateral.
   B. The position of the saphenous nerve is always medial.
   C. The position of the saphenous nerve is lateral in the adductor canal and medial in the lower third of the thigh.
   D. The position of the saphenous nerve is medial in the adductor canal and lateral in the lower third of the thigh.

72. All of the following statements are true regarding the boundaries of paravertebral space EXCEPT:

   A. The boundaries of the three-sided wedge—posterior, medial boundary, and anterolateral—extend caudally and cephalad, as the segmental spaces communicate up and down.
   B. The PVS is bounded posteriorly by transverse processes and the rib heads.
   C. The medial boundary is the vertebral body, the intervertebral disks, and the intervertebral foramen at each level.
   D. The anterolateral boundary is the parietal pleura.
   E. Laterally, the space tapers and closes.

73. All of the following are indications of thoracic paravertebral block EXCEPT:

   A. Thoracic surgery
   B. Breast surgery
   C. Cholecystectomy and upper abdominal surgeries
   D Knee surgery
   E. Renal and ureteric surgery

74. Which statement about the thoracic paravertebral block contraindications is MOST likely true?

   A. Kyphoscoliosis is an absolute contraindication for thoracic paravertebral block.
   B. Thoracic paravertebral block is not contraindicated in a patient with severe coagulopathy.
   C. Infection at the site of needle insertion is an absolute contraindication.
   D. Paravertebral or pleural space infections are not contraindications for the block.

75. All of the following are advantages of paravertebral block (PVB) compared to epidural block EXCEPT:

   A. PVB is associated with less urinary retention.
   B. PVB is associated with less PONV.
   C. PVB is associated with less hypotension.
   D. PVB had fewer pulmonary complications.
   E. All of the above

76. The following statement is true or false: The spinal nerves in this space are devoid of a fascial sheath, making them susceptible to local anesthetics.

   A. True
   B. False

77. Which statement about the local anesthetic spread in the PVS is MOST likely true?

    A. The PVS communicates with spaces above and below.

    B. Fifteen to 20 mL injections cover approximately four dermatomes.

    C. Accumulation of bupivacaine occurs during continuous paravertebral infusion without clinical signs of toxicity.

    D. The addition of 5 mcg/mL epinephrine to ropivacaine significantly delays its systemic absorption.

    E. The absorption of ropivacaine after TPVB is described by rapid and slow absorption phases.

    F. All of the above

78. In the classic PVB landmark approach, which of the following is MOST likely true?

    A. Needle insertion is 2.5 to 3 cm lateral to the cephalad edge of the spinous process.

    B. The needle is advanced perpendicular to the skin until the transverse process is contacted.

    C. The needle is advanced 1 to 1.5 cm.

    D. A pop or click may be felt just prior to entry into the PVS.

    E. All of the above

79. In this ultrasound image from the thoracic paravertebral region, please identify the following:

    A. Thoracic paravertebral space

    B. Pleura

    C. Paraspinal muscles

    D. Superior costotransverse ligament

    E. Lung

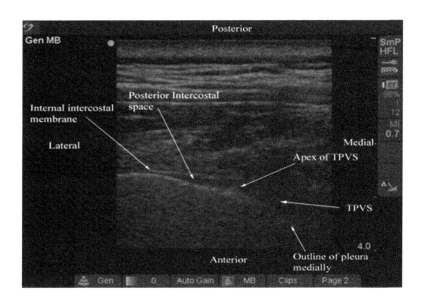

80. The lumbar plexus is formed by which nerve roots?

    A. Anterior divisions of L1 to L4 nerve roots
    B. Posterior divisions of L1 to L4 nerve roots
    C. Anterior divisions of L1 to S1 nerve roots
    D. Posterior divisions of L1 to S1 nerve roots

81. The lumbar plexus lies within which muscle?

    A. Erector spinae
    B. Psoas major
    C. Quadratus lumborum
    D. Iliacus

82. Which of the following nerve blocks can be used for most effective postoperative analgesia following total hip arthroplasty?

    A. Lumbar plexus block
    B. TAP block
    C. Obturator nerve block
    D. Peroneal nerve block

83. Which of the following landmarks are used for a classic Winnie's approach for lumbar plexus block?

    A. Greater trochanter, ischial tuberosity, and spinous process
    B. Intercristal line, spinous process, and posterior superior iliac spine
    C. Intercristal line, sacral hiatus, and spinous process
    D. Intercristal line, greater trochanter, and sacral hiatus

84. Which muscle is lateral to the sciatic nerve when it reaches the popliteal fossa?

    A. Semimembranosus muscle
    B. Semitendinosus muscle
    C. Gastrocnemius muscle
    D. Biceps femoris muscle

85. A patient is scheduled for an Achilles tendon repair and has a history of a femoral-popliteal bypass. On ultrasound, the typical vascular structures you use to orient yourself are not distinct, and it is difficult for you to confirm the location of the sciatic nerve due to scar tissue. You decide to use the nerve stimulator simultaneously with the ultrasound. When using nerve stimulation to identify the proper location for performing the popliteal block, you know you are in the correct location if your stimulation results in:

    A. Plantar flexion
    B. Dorsiflexion
    C. Eversion
    D. Inversion
    E. Paresthesias of the medial lower leg
    F. All of the above
    G. A and D
    H. B and C

86. The common peroneal nerve is larger than the posterior tibial nerve.

    A. True
    B. False

87. What is the dumbbell sign?

    A. An ultrasound artifact
    B. When the biceps femoris, semimembranosus, and semitendinosus tendons are accentuated upon flexion of the knee
    C. The merging of the common peroneal and posterior tibial nerves
    D. When the block achieves sensory blockade without motor blockade

88. You decide to perform a popliteal fossa block with the patient in the supine position because the patient has an external fixation device at the ankle. You insert your needle and notice that it is a few centimeters inferior to the sciatic nerve. In order to redirect your needle closer to the nerve, you:

    A. Lift your hand upward to direct the needle more inferior and deep

    B. Lift your hand upward to direct the needle more inferior and superficial (toward the interface between the skin and the ultrasound probe)

    C. Move your hand downward to direct the needle more superior and deep

    D. Move your hand downward to direct the needle more superior and superficial

89. The surgeon is planning to perform a below knee amputation (BKA) on a patient without using a tourniquet. This patient has multiple comorbidities including congestive heart failure, coronary artery disease, stroke, and chronic kidney disease; therefore you decide to perform a surgical block on the patient in order to avoid general anesthesia. You plan to perform a:

    A. Single-shot popliteal block and adductor canal block using ropivacaine 0.2%

    B. Single-shot popliteal block and adductor canal block using ropivacaine 0.5%

    C. Single-shot subgluteal sciatic nerve block and femoral nerve block using ropivacaine 0.2%

    D. Single-shot subgluteal sciatic nerve block and femoral nerve block using ropivacaine 0.5%

90. Which of the following is NOT true regarding the sciatic nerve?

    A. It is derived from the sacral plexus.

    B. It exits the pelvis from the lesser sciatic notch.

    C. It lies deep to the gluteus maximus.

    D. It runs between the greater trochanter and the ischial tuberosity.

91. During an ultrasound-guided transgluteal sciatic nerve block, all of the following statements are true EXCEPT:

    A. The bony landmarks used are ischial tuberosity and greater trochanter.

    B. The use of a nerve stimulator improves the success rate of the block.

    C. A high-frequency probe is preferred for deeper penetration.

    D. The nerve is most commonly located in the middle of the bony landmarks used.

92. Which of the following statement is FALSE regarding the sciatic nerve?

    A. It is the largest peripheral nerve in the body.

    B. Combined with saphenous nerve block, it provides complete analgesia for foot surgery.

    C. It arises from the nerve roots L4 to S2.

    D. The landmarks used in ultrasound-guided blocks are the greater trochanter and sacral hiatus.

93. Regarding the anterior approach (as described by Beck) for sciatic nerve block, all of the following are true EXCEPT:

    A. The anterior superior iliac spine and pubic tubercle are landmarks.

    B. The greater trochanter and pubic tubercle are landmarks.

    C. Anesthesia of the posterior aspect of the thigh may be missed.

    D. A needle inserted too laterally can injure the blood vessels.

94. All of the following are true regarding the ultrasound-guided anterior approach to sciatic nerve block EXCEPT:

    A. The use of a low-frequency probe is preferred.
    B. In patients with coagulopathy, it is preferably avoided.
    C. Slight internal rotation of the thigh helps to give a better view of the anatomy.
    D. It is ideal for patients who cannot be placed laterally.

95. Regarding the ultrasound-guided transgluteal approach to sciatic nerve block, all of the following statements are true EXCEPT:

    A. It is indicated for surgery on the tibia, ankle and foot.
    B. The landmarks used are the greater trochanter and the posterior superior iliac spine.
    C. Combined with a lumbar plexus block, anesthesia of the entire lower extremity can be achieved.
    D. In contrast to common belief, it is a relatively easy block to perform, with a high success rate.

96. What are the most sensitive signs of accidental intravascular injection of local anesthetics in caudal blocks in pediatric patients?

    A. An increase in the T wave amplitude greater than 25% of baseline; ST segment changes
    B. An increase in the heart rate greater than 10 beats per minute
    C. An increase in the systolic blood pressure greater than 15 mm Hg
    D. Hypotension

97. What are the anatomical differences between pediatric and adult patients in the caudal and dural sac level?

    A. The spinal cord ends at the L1 level in neonates and at the L3 level in adults.
    B. The dural sac ends at the S1 level in adults and the S3 level in neonates.
    C. The CSF volume/body weight ratio is higher in adults than in pediatric patients.
    D. When performing a spinal block in a pediatric patient, the interspace L1 to L2 is preferred to minimize the risk of spinal cord injury.

98. How would you manage an accidental injection of local intravascular anesthetic that causes HD changes?

    A. Propofol
    B. Midazolam
    C. Intralipids
    D. Benadryl

99. What fascia is pierced in performing a penile block?

    A. Fascia iliaca
    B. Fascia lata
    C. Buck's fascia
    D. No fascia

100. Identify what kind of block is in the following ultrasound picture.

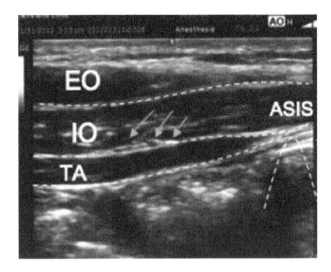

A. Transversus abdominis plane block
B. Rectus sheath block
C. Quadratus lumborum block
D. Ilioinguinal/iliohypogastric block

101. Which of the following is true regarding the incidence of neurological injury?

A. The use of ultrasound guidance has decreased the reported frequency of long-term neurological symptoms.
B. Data confirms that proximal nerve blocks are riskier than distal approaches.
C. The incidence of injury after neuraxial blockade is extremely low, and injuries are rarely permanent.
D. Postoperative neurological symptoms after peripheral nerve block are common but rarely result in permanent injury.

102. Which of the following is not a risk factor for neuraxial injury (hematoma, infection, direct spinal cord injury)?

A. Epidural technique as compared to subarachnoid technique
B. Associated coagulation abnormalities
C. Concurrent spinal stenosis
D. Obstetric procedures

103. Which of the following is not a risk factor contributing to perioperative peripheral nerve injury?

A. Epidural and general anesthetics
B. Peripheral nerve block
C. Intrafascicular injection of local anesthetic
D. Tourniquet

104. Which of the following orthopedic surgeries are correctly paired with the most commonly associated nerve injured?

A. Shoulder surgery—radial nerve
B. Elbow surgery—musculocutaneous nerve
C. Hip surgery—superior gluteal nerve
D. Knee surgery—common peroneal nerve

105. Which of the following is true with regard to blood pressure control during neuraxial anesthesia?

A. Local anesthetics, adjuvants, epinephrine, and phenylephrine may adversely affect spinal cord blood flow.
B. The accepted cerebral lower limit of autoregulation for spinal cord blood flow is 50 mm Hg mean arterial pressure (MAP).
C. The recommendation is to maintain blood pressure at least within 20% to 30% of baseline MAP during neuraxial anesthesia.
D. Periods of severe and prolonged hypotension are strongly associated with sustained cerebral or spinal cord ischemia.

106. Which of the following is true regarding chlorhexidine?

   A. Chlorhexidine solution should be allowed to completely dry on skin before needle placement.

   B. A retrospective cohort study showed an increased risk of arachnoiditis with the use of chlorhexidine.

   C. Chlorhexidine is inferior to iodine-alcohol as an antiseptic agent.

   D. Chlorhexidine should be placed alongside block trays and instruments.

107. Which of the following is true with regard to performing neuraxial techniques in anesthetized or deeply sedated patients?

   A. Ultrasound guidance has been shown to reduce the risk of neuraxial injury in patients under general anesthesia or deep sedation.

   B. Placing peripheral and neuraxial nerve blocks in an anesthetized adult does not increase injury rate.

   C. Neuraxial techniques should be performed under general anesthesia or deep sedation in pediatric patients.

   D. Paresthesia and pain on injection of local anesthetic are consistent warning signs of needle contact with the spinal cord.

108. Which of the following is true with regard to prevention of peripheral nerve injury?

   A. Ultrasound can detect intraneural injection.

   B. Paresthesia during needle advancement or on injection of local anesthetic is highly predictive of peripheral nerve injury.

   C. Data supports the use of ultrasound as the superior technique to reduce the likelihood of peripheral nerve injury as compared to peripheral nerve stimulator and injection pressure monitoring.

   D. Current ultrasound technology has adequate resolution to discern between an interfascicular and intrafascicular injection.

109. Regarding performing regional anesthesia on patients with diabetes and diabetic polyneuropathy, which of the following is false?

   A. Ensuring addition of adjuvant epinephrine is important.

   B. Consideration should be given to limiting local anesthetic concentration/dose.

   C. Although current research is still limited, a small number of clinical studies do attest to higher peripheral nerve block success rates in diabetic patients.

   D. Diabetic nerves are less sensitive to electrical stimulation, which theoretically increases the risk of intraneural needle placement.

110. What is the incidence of peripheral neuropathy development in patients who receive neurotoxic chemotherapeutic agents?

   A. Less than 25%

   B. 30% to 40%

   C. 50% to 75%

   D. 100%

111. Regarding previous spine surgery, which of the following is false?

- **A.** Under most circumstances, spinal anesthesia has a higher success rate than epidural techniques.
- **B.** Neuraxial anesthetics are not contraindicated.
- **C.** Interventional pain medicine techniques are not contraindicated.
- **D.** These patients are at a higher risk for developing neurological deficits when undergoing spinal anesthesia; therefore risk versus benefit must be analyzed when deciding between general and regional anesthesia.

112. The risk of iatrogenic spinal cord trauma can be completely eliminated by:

- **A.** Needle placement through the L3 to L4 vertebral interspace
- **B.** Expecting resistance prior to entering the epidural space during midline approach to the neuraxis
- **C.** Expecting uniform dorsoventral dimension of the posterior epidural space along the entire vertebral column
- **D.** None of the above

113. Spinal cord perfusion pressure can potentially be diminished by all of the following EXCEPT:

- **A.** An increased systemic to cerebrospinal fluid pressure gradient
- **B.** Excessive volumes of local anesthetics
- **C.** Chronic morphine administration via intrathecal delivery systems
- **D.** Surgical procedures performed in extreme lateral flexion in patients with severe spinal stenosis

114. In a morbidly obese patient with known extradural tumor at the T7 vertebral level, awaiting thoracotomy for pneumonectomy:

- **A.** Radiologic evaluation of the neuraxis should be considered to better characterize the extent of the tumor.
- **B.** Epidural catheter placement and bolusing local anesthetic via the catheter can always be safely performed.
- **C.** Significant and prolonged systemic hypotension is preferred to minimize blood loss.
- **D.** Surgical positioning is not relevant as long as it provides excellent exposure of the operative field.

115. Which of the following is associated with an increased risk of complications after a neuraxial blockade?

- **A.** Hypertrophy of the ligamentum flavum
- **B.** Nonneutral patient positioning
- **C.** Surface landmarks that are difficult to appreciate
- **D.** All of the above

116. In normotensive, unanesthetized adults, the lower limit of spinal cord autoregulation is approximately:

- **A.** 50 to 55 mm Hg
- **B.** 55 to 60 mm Hg
- **C.** 60 to 65 mm Hg
- **D.** 65 to 70 mm Hg

117. Which of the following statements regarding spinal cord perfusion is true?

A. Preoperative hypertension is an accurate predictor of the lower limit of spinal cord autoregulation.

B. Intrathecal epinephrine adversely affects the spinal cord blood flow.

C. Sickle cell disease may increase the risk of spinal cord ischemia.

D. Prolonged sensory and motor blockade after neuraxial anesthesia or analgesia is a sign of residual local anesthetic effect; therefore, no further workup is necessary.

118. Regarding the safety of performing a neuraxial blockade on patients taking oral anticoagulants, which of the following statements is INCORRECT?

A. Dabigatran should be discontinued at least 48 hours before neuraxial injection.

B. Prasugrel should be discontinued at least 7 to 10 days before neuraxial injection.

C. In patients taking fondaparinux, if a neuraxial technique has to be performed, single-needle neuraxial technique is recommended, and an indwelling catheter placement should be avoided.

D. In patients on recent bivalirudin therapy, an anticoagulant effect should be pharmacologically reversed prior to performance of neuraxial techniques.

119. The risk of arachnoiditis resulting from the use of chlorhexidine as a skin disinfectant is minimal when:

A. Chlorhexidine is allowed to completely dry on skin before needle placement.

B. There is temporal and physical separation of the block tray from chlorhexidine.

C. Care is taken to avoid needle or catheter contamination from chlorhexidine.

D. All of the above

120. The risk of spinal hematoma formation, relative to patients with no preexisting coagulopathy and atraumatic needle placement, is the greatest in patients:

A. With no preexisting coagulopathy, after traumatic needle placement

B. Receiving heparin longer than 1 hour after atraumatic needle placement

C. On aspirin and receiving heparin longer than 1 hour after needle placement

D. On heparin anticoagulation longer than 1 hour after traumatic needle placement

121. When administered intrathecally, clonidine provides an analgesic effect by:

A. Binding to α_2 receptors in the substantia gelatinosa in the spinal cord

B. Binding to the intermediolateral column in the spinal cord

C. Interacting with excitatory AMPA and inhibitory GABA receptors

D. All of the above

122. The incidence of postdural puncture headache decreases with:

A. Decreasing age

B. Increasing age

C. Needle insertion perpendicular to the dural fibers

D. Identifying the epidural space by the loss of resistance to air as opposed to loss of resistance to saline technique

Answers

1. **(C)** Coagulopathy is a relative contraindication for TAP block. The TAP block depends on the spread of local anesthetic in a large plane; hence it is a high-volume, low-concentration block. It is used as an adjunct for anterior abdominal wall incisions/drains. It does not provide adequate analgesia as a sole anesthetic as it does not block the visceral component. Also, the spread of local anesthetic in the TAP plane depends on the volume and site of injection. Saline can be used to hydrodissect and identify the TAP plane with-out wasting LA volume while seeking the ideal place to deposit the LA.

2. **(D)** The anterolateral abdominal wall is innervated by the anterior rami of the lower six thoracic nerves (T7 to T12) and the first lumbar nerve (L1). The nerves lie in the fascial plane between the internal oblique and the transversus abdominis muscles. Injection of local anesthetic within the TAP can provide unilateral analgesia to the skin, muscles, and parietal peritoneum of the anterior abdominal wall from T7 to L1 depending on the volume and site of injection.

3. **(C)** The Petit triangle is situated between the lower costal margin and the iliac crest. It is bound anteriorly by the external oblique muscle and posteriorly by the latissimus dorsi muscle. This technique relies on feeling double pops as the needle traverses the external oblique and internal oblique muscles. A blunt needle will make the loss of resistance more appreciable.

4. **(C)** The transversus abdominis plane can be traced from its insertion to the linea alba (lateral to rectus abdominis) and is best viewed in the lateral part of the abdomen. The TAP block provides analgesia to the abdominal wall but provides no visceral analgesia. It should be used in combination with an oral or intravenous analgesia. Observing the spread of local anesthetic is essential, ensuring the needle tip is in the transversus abdominis plane. The in-plane technique is ideal to visualize the needle tip and facilitates the identification of the TAP plane.

5. **(B)** Subcostal TAP was described by Hebbard and associates for providing analgesia after upper abdominal surgery. The subcostal TAP is a neurofascial plane between the rectus abdominis and the transversus abdominis muscles. Deposition of LA in this plane has shown to block dermatomes T6 to T10 with occasional spread to T12, definitely sparing the L1 dermatome. A TAP block does not cause sympathetic block.

6. **(C)** The anterolateral abdominal wall is innervated by the anterior rami of the lower six thoracic nerves (T7 to T12) and the first lumbar nerve (L1). The muscles of the anterolateral abdominal wall are external oblique, internal oblique, and transversus abdominis muscles. The external oblique muscle is the largest of the three muscles. The nerves lie in the fascial plane between the internal oblique and the transversus abdominis muscles.

7. **(A)** This is a chronic pain patient who will need multimodal analgesia to manage postoperative pain. In view of the previous history of pulmonary embolism and Lovenox administration, an epidural and paravertebral block may not be the safest modes of analgesia. The rectus sheath block provides analgesia for midline incisions but will not be effective for ileostomy.

8. **(B)** The TAP plane is the fascial plane between the internal oblique muscle and the transversus abdominis muscle. The order of structures in the abdominal wall are skin, fat, external oblique, internal oblique, transversus abdominis, and peritoneum.

9. **(D)** Posterior TAP blocks will provide analgesia for lower abdominal surgeries. For a large midline laparotomy incision, local anesthetic should be deposited bilaterally in the subcostal TAP planes and the Petit triangle. Catheter placement in the TAP plane is relatively easy and has been shown to be an effective means of pain relief.

10. **(C)** Amide local anesthetics are lidocaine, mepivacaine, and prilocaine, and they all are metabolized by cytochrome P450 enzymes in the liver. Ester, like procaine, is metabolized by pseudocholinesterase.

11. **(B)** Exparel should not be mixed with any other local anesthetic, though it can be diluted with normal saline.

12. **(A)** Manifestations of local anesthetic toxicity typically appear 1 to 5 minutes after the injection. Classically, systemic toxicity begins with symptoms of CNS excitement, such as circumoral and/or tongue numbness, metallic taste, lightheadedness, dizziness, visual and auditory disturbances (difficulty focusing and tinnitus), disorientation, and drowsiness. With higher doses, initial CNS excitation is often followed by a rapid CNS depression, with the following features: muscle twitching, convulsions, unconsciousness, coma, respiratory depression and arrest, cardiovascular depression, and collapse.

13. **(A, B, and C)** These three are part of checklist for the treatment of local anesthetic systemic toxicity. Option "D" is incorrect. Recommendation is to double the infusion rate to 0.5 mL/kg/min if the blood pressure remains low.

14. **(E)** All the statements are true.

15. **(A)** Amide local anesthetics (LAs) are metabolized in the liver by cytochrome P450 enzymes. These enzymes reach adult activity level by 9 months to 1 year. Therefore, neonates and infants have a higher serum-free fraction of amide LAs and are more prone to develop toxicity.

16. **(B)** Direct cardiac toxicity is due to a prolonged blockade of the sodium channels in the cardiac conduction system, resulting in a profound decrease in ventricular conduction velocity. The susceptibility to cardiac toxicity is amplified by increased heart rates.

Neonates and infants are more sensitive than adults to cardiotoxicity induced by amide LAs because of their higher baseline heart rates.

17. (C) Neonates have a larger total volume of CSF compared to adults (4 mL/kg compared to 2 mL/kg, respectively). In addition, 50% of the total CSF volume is in the spinal portion of the subarachnoid space compared to only 25% of the total CSF volume in adults. Also, neonates have a more rapid turnover of CSF than do adults. As a result, neonates require larger doses of LAs for spinal anesthesia, and the duration of the spinal block is shorter.

18. (A) Chloroprocaine is increasingly used to provide continuous epidural infusion for post-operative pain control in neonates. It is rapidly metabolized by cholinesterases, with an elimination half-life of a few minutes. Although neonates have a reduced level of plasma esterases compared to the level in adults, this is clinically insignificant. Therefore the incidence of systemic toxicity is rare, and the risk of accumulation is minimal. This safety profile allows better analgesia in neonates as it allows the use of higher infusion rates and thus wider dermatomal coverage compared to amide LAs.

19. (A) The interscalene block is most successfully performed utilizing the posterior triangle, which lies between the posterior border of the sternocleidomastoid and trapezius muscles, at the level of the sixth and seventh cervical vertebrae.

20. (D) The dorsal scapular and long thoracic nerves appear as hyperechoic structures with a hypoechoic center found in the middle scalene less than 1 cm posterior to the brachial plexus.

21. (A) Injury to the dorsal scapular nerve is characterized by a dull ache along the medial border of the scapulae along with weakness/hypotrophy of the rhomboid and levator scapulae muscles.

22. (C) Injury to the long thoracic nerve typically presents as chronic pain of the shoulder as well as weakness of the serratus anterior muscle, manifesting as the classic "winged scapula" when a patient pushes an outstretched hand against a wall.

23. (C) The most common complication associated with an interscalene block is involvement of the ipsilateral phrenic nerve; thus caution must be taking with patients who have limited pulmonary function.

24. (D) Practically, using ultrasound in the supraclavicular approach for the brachial plexus, the trunks and the divisions appear as a compact group of nerves (bunch of grapes) lying superior and posterior to the artery.

25. (C) The catheter is usually inserted superior to the subclavian artery in the case of shoulder surgery or in the corner pocket between the artery and first rib in the case of hand surgery. The correct position of the catheter can be confirmed under ultrasound by injecting a local anesthetic or 1 mL of air into the catheter and observing its distribution in relation to the plexus.

26. (A) An injury to the suprascapular nerve following a supraclavicular block is usually presented by severe shoulder pain followed by weakness in supraspinatus and infraspinatus muscles. To avoid this complication, try not to inject above the plexus to avoid exposing the nerve to a toxic high concentration of local anesthetics. In addition, avoiding injection above the plexus might decrease the incidence of phrenic nerve palsy after the block.

27. (E) To avoid this complication, try not to inject above the plexus to avoid exposing the nerve to a toxic high concentration of local anesthetics. In addition, avoiding injection above the plexus might decrease the incidence of phrenic nerve palsy after the block.

28. (B) The brachial plexus in the supraclavicular region is composed mainly of three trunks: superior, middle, and inferior. These trunks pass across the upper surface of the first rib, where they lie posterior and superior to the subclavian artery. The trunks then divide into anterior and posterior divisions behind the clavicle.

29. (A) Try to examine the anterior chest wall by ultrasound after every supraclavicular block to confirm the absence of pneumothorax by visualizing the intact pleura (sliding sign).

30. (C) The block can be used for shoulder, elbow, or hand surgery; however, it can miss the lower portion of the brachial plexus, thus sparing the ulnar nerve distribution of the medial side of the hand.

31. (B) Local anesthetic toxicity typically occurs due to inadvertent intravascular or intrathecal injection or an excessive dosage leading to elevated blood concentrations of the drug. Initial signs/symptoms of local anesthetic toxicity include lightheadedness, dizziness, and numbness of the tongue. Further CNS excitation can occur, manifesting as visual or auditory disturbances, shivering or muscle twitching, and ultimately, seizure (generalized tonic-clonic seizures). Even higher plasma drug levels will lead to cardiovascular collapse.

32. (D) An axillary block can provide excellent pain coverage for surgeries on the midarm down to the elbow, on elbow surgeries, and on wrist and hand surgeries. An axillary block will not provide pain control for shoulder surgeries. An interscalene block and a supraclavicular block would provide excellent pain control for shoulder surgeries.

33. (A) The median nerve originates from both the medial and lateral cords. It provides motor branches to the flexors of the hand and wrist. It provides sensory innervation to the palmar surface of the first, second, third digits, and the lateral half of the fourth digit.

34. (E) A hematoma can occur during an axillary block, especially if the patient was on an anticoagulant or if there are multiple needle punctures to the veins or axillary artery.

The most common cause of local anesthetic systemic toxicity during an axillary block is inadvertent intravascular injection. To avoid systemic toxicity during an axillary block, avoid fast forceful injection of local anesthetic, perform careful frequent aspiration during the injection, and adjust the dose and volume of local anesthetic injected in frail and elderly patients.

35. (B) Under ultrasound, the musculocutaneous nerve has a characteristic appearance of a hypoechoic flattened oval with a bright hyperechoic rim.

36. (A)

37. (B)

38. (C)

39. (D)

40. (B) Infraclavicular blocks typically occur at the level of the cords of the brachial plexus. The axillary approach blocks the terminal nerves. The interscalene approach blocks the roots (or trunks), whereas the supraclavicular approach typically blocks the divisions.

41. (C) The infraclavicular approach to the brachial plexus occurs in the axilla. In this space, the subclavian artery has become the axillary artery. The axillary artery lies superior (cephalad) to the axillary vein. In this image, a branch of the axillary artery is noted running superior to the main artery as well.

42. (B) The brachial plexus and axillary vessels lie just deep to the fascia of the pectoralis minor muscle. It is critical to deposit local anesthetic deep to this fascia or the block will fail.

43. (D) The intercostobrachial nerve arises from T2 and is not anesthetized by any approach to the brachial plexus. It may be blocked by subcutaneous infiltration of local anesthetic under the ventral side of the proximal arm.

44. (D) The cords of the brachial plexus surround the axillary artery. With the left side of the screen oriented cephalad, the lateral, posterior, and medial cords are often found at 9 to 10 o'clock, 6 to 7 o'clock, and 4 to 5 o'clock relative to the artery, respectively.

45. (A) The axillary vessels and brachial plexus often lie deep to the clavicle. Abducting the arm and flexing the elbow will often bring the structures caudally, allowing ultrasound visualization. More medial approaches are not recommended due to proximity to the pleura.

46. (B) Although all the structures can be found in a typical transverse scan of the inguinal region, the femoral nerve is typically superficial to the iliopsoas muscle and lateral to the femoral artery. The fascia lata is superficial and can be found in the subcutaneous layer.

47. (A) Posteriorly, the base of the femoral triangle is formed by the pectineus, iliopsoas, and adductor longus muscles. Part of the adductor longus muscle also forms the medial border of the triangle, whereas the superior and lateral borders are formed by the inguinal ligament and medial border of the sartorius muscle, respectively.

48. (C) A twitch of the sartorius muscle can be commonly seen when using nerve stimulation for localization of the femoral nerve. A band-like contraction of the thigh without movement of the patella is often how sartorius muscle stimulation manifests and why it can be mistaken for stimulation of the femoral nerve. Sartorius muscle stimulation is not a reliable response because the nerve branches to the sartorius muscle off of the femoral nerve may be outside of the femoral sheath.

49. (D) Inguinal lymph nodes also appear hyperechoic and can be mistaken for the femoral nerve in a short-axis view. Scanning proximally and distally distinguishes the two structures because a nerve is a continuous structure, whereas a lymph node can only be seen in a discrete location.

50. (B) The femoral nerve is superficial to the iliopsoas muscle and is deep to or covered by the fascia iliaca. Occasionally, the nerve can be found between layers of the fascia iliaca. The transversalis fascia contributes to the formation of the inguinal ligament and extends to form the separate vascular fascia of the femoral artery and vein. The fascia lata is superficial to the fascia iliaca.

51. (C) A higher-frequency transducer (8 to 14 MHz) produces the best image resolution for superficial structures. This is at the expense of a limited depth of penetration. A lower-frequency transducer (less than 7 MHz) is therefore required for imaging deeper structures. The femoral nerve is typically visualized at a shallow depth, which obviates the need for a lower-frequency transducer. Curvilinear ultrasound probes often generate lower-frequency waves, and as a result, produce images with poorer visibility due to the lower resolution.

52. (A) The obturator nerve arises form the anterior primary rami of L2 to L4 nerve roots.

53. (C) The obturator nerve divides into anterior and posterior divisions. The anterior division lies between adductor longus and adductor brevis muscles.

54. (B) The anterior division provides sensory supply to the medial thigh and supplies articular branches to the medial hip joint.

55. (A) The posterior division of the obturator nerve supplies articular branches to the medial knee joint.

56. (C) The adductors of the legs are supplied by the obturator nerve, and it exits the pelvis through the obturator foramen.

57. **(C)** The QL block produces a more extensive, predictable, and posterior spread of local anesthetic, similar to that seen with the landmark TAP block in that there is subsequent extension into the thoracic paravertebral space. A QL block results in a wider sensory blockade compared to TAP block (T7 to L1 for QL block vs. T10 to T12 for the TAP block). Ultrasound-guided TAP blocks not are able to produce a sensory level above the umbilicus consistently unless you add a subcostal injection. An ultrasound-guided QL block has been introduced and shown to result in consistent coverage of at least T8 rostrally and L1 caudally. Moreover, a QL block has the potential to provide some visceral analgesia, considering its spread to paravertebral and potentially epidural spaces. Potential advantages of QL over TAP are wider dermatomal coverage (T6 to L1), potential coverage of the pelvic and abdominal visceral pain, and a longer duration.

58. **(A)** K

(B) N

(C) J

(D) M

(E) D

The quadratus lumborum muscle is a muscle of the posterior abdominal wall, lying deep inside the abdomen and dorsal to the iliopsoas. It originates from the medial half of the iliac crest and inserts into the lower medial border of the last rib (twelfth), and by four small tendons from the apices of the transverse processes of the upper four lumbar vertebrae. The quadratus lumborum assists in producing lateral flexion of the lumbar spine. The ventral rami pass between the QL and its anterior fascia. The QL muscle tendons attached to the lumbar transverse process under ultrasound usually look like a small boat hooked to a stick (transverse process); the psoas muscle looks like water under the QL muscle and is usually hyperechoic at this level because of its intramuscular fibrous tendon structure and because it is surrounded by thick fibrous thoracolumbar fascia (TLF). The TLF consists of both aponeurotic and fascial connective tissue. Its most important function is providing a retinaculum for paraspinal musculature in the lumbar region. It consists of three layers: anterior, middle, and posterior. Anterior to the middle layer, the quadratus lumborum is situated, which is separated from the psoas by the anterior layer, that courses between them. The posterior and middle layers of the thoracolumbar fascia fuse laterally to form the lateral raphe, a weave of connective tissue that then joins with two abdominal muscles—the transversus abdominis and internal oblique. These muscles wrap around to the front, surround the rectus abdominis, and merge at the linea alba. The four lumbar arteries, one on each side, arise from the posterior surface of the aorta at the level of L1 to L4 vertebrae; they course posterior to the psoas major muscle and are covered by the psoas major muscle and the sympathetic trunk. Between the transverse processes of the vertebrae, each lumbar artery divides into a dorsal and an abdominal branch. The abdominal branches of the lumbar arteries run laterally behind the quadratus lumborum muscle, and then forward between the abdominal muscles to supply the abdominal wall. The lowest branch sometimes passes in front of the quadratus lumborum. The QL blocks the lateral cutaneous branches

(LCBs) of the thoracoabdominal nerves (T6 to L1), which arise proximal to the angle of the rib and emerge through the overlying muscles in the midaxillary line to supply the skin of the lateral thorax, the abdomen, the iliac crest, and the upper thigh. The subcostal and iliohypogastric nerves pass deep over the anterior surface of the quadratus lumborum muscle. The QL blocks will block both the anterior and the lateral branches of the thoracoabdominal nerves.

59. (A) The quadratus lumborum muscle is a muscle of the posterior abdominal wall lying deep inside the abdomen and dorsal to the iliopsoas. The QL muscle originates from the medial half of the iliac crest and inserts into the lower medial border of the last rib (twelfth), and by four small tendons from the apices of the transverse processes of the upper four lumbar vertebrae. The quadratus lumborum assists in producing lateral flexion of the lumbar spine. The ventral rami pass between the QL and its anterior fascia.

60. (D) The QL block can provide unilateral analgesia and can preserve bladder and lower limb motor function. It also avoids the sympathectomy and hemodynamic instability following the cardiovascular effects of epidural block. A QL block can be performed in sedated and ventilated patients.

61. (E)

62. (E)

63. (B)

64. (A)

65. (B)

Explanation for questions 62 through 65:

QL indications: Unfortunately without strong evidence, it is based on case reports and experience. This block shares the same indications as the transversus abdominis plane (TAP) block, in addition to some surgeries with the incision above the umbilicus, and as a component of multimodal postoperative analgesia for a wide variety of abdominal procedures (any type of operation that requires intraabdominal visceral pain to be covered plus abdominal wall incisions as high as T6). The QL block is conducive to placement of a continuous catheter for:

- Large bowel resection, open/laparoscopic appendectomy and cholecystectomy
- Cesarean section, total abdominal hysterectomy
- Open prostatectomy, renal transplant surgery, nephrectomy, abdominoplasty, and iliac crest bone graft
- Ileostomy
- Exploratory laparotomy, bilateral blocks for midline incisions

Complications of the QL block are related to the lack of anatomical understanding and needle expertise. It is possible to puncture intraabdominal structures such as the kidney, liver, and spleen. Extra caution should be taken especially for the right-sided block, as the right kidney is slightly lower than the left kidney and appears smaller when seen with ultrasound. Transient femoral nerve palsy has been noticed in some patients and attributed to the spread of medication to the lumber plexus and tracking of medication under the fascia iliaca. In bilateral blocks with high volume, systemic local anesthetic toxicity should be considered.

66. **(D)** The adductor canal is also called the subsartorial or Hunter's canal. This is an aponeurotic tunnel in the middle third of the thigh, extending from the apex of the femoral triangle to the opening in the adductor magnus.

67. **(A)** The short-axis ultrasound image of the adductor canal at the midthigh usually shows the sartorius muscle and the saphenous nerve (posterior division) as hyperechoic structures lateral to the artery and anterior to the vein. The vastus medialis muscle lies laterally to the saphenous nerve, whereas the adductor longus and adductor magnus muscles are on its medial side.

68. **(D)** The saphenous nerve is a terminal branch of femoral nerve, which provides sensory coverage to skin in front of knee and the medial side of the leg and feet.

69. **(C)** A and B represent superficial skin and subcutaneous tissue; D represents vastus medialis muscle.

70. **(A)**

71. **(C)** The saphenous nerve is located lateral to the superficial femoral artery in the adductor canal and then crosses over the superficial femoral artery anteriorly just proximal of the lower end of the adductor magnus muscle and runs medially alongside the superficial femoral artery until emerging from the canal with the saphenous branch of the descending genicular artery.

72. **(E)** The thoracic paravertebral space (TPVS), when viewed in transverse cross-section, is triangular-shaped (dashed triangle in figure below). The base is formed by the posterolateral aspect of the vertebral body/intervertebral disks/intervertebral foramina/articular processes. The anterolateral border is formed by the parietal pleura, whereas the posterior border is formed by the superior costotransverse ligament. The TPVS contains mainly fatty tissue and is traversed by the intercostal or spinal nerves, intercostal vessels, dorsal rami, rami communicantes, and the sympathetic chain. The spinal nerves do not have a fascial sheath in the TPVS, which explains their susceptibility to local anesthetic blockade. The spinal nerves with their ganglia were found within subendothoracic and posteromedial (SETC) fascia, whereas the sympathetic ganglia were consistently located within the extrapleural and anterolateral (EPC) fascia. The boundaries of the three-sided wedge—posterior, medial, and anterolateral—extend caudally and cephalad, as the segmental spaces communicate up and down. The PVS is bounded posteriorly by

transverse processes, the rib heads, and the ligaments that travel between the adjacent transverse processes and ribs. The medial boundary is the vertebral body, the intervertebral disks, and the intervertebral foramen at each level. The anterolateral boundary is the parietal pleura. Laterally, the space tapers as it communicates with the intercostal space.

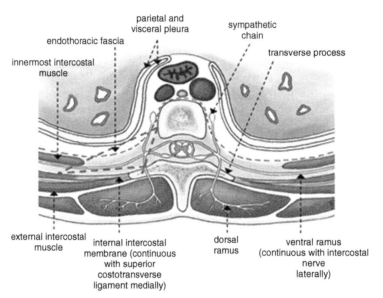

73. **(D)** The TPVB offers several technical and clinical advantages and is indicated for anesthesia and analgesia when the afferent pain input is predominantly unilateral from the chest and/or abdomen. Bilateral TPVB has also been used perioperatively during thoracic, major abdominal vascular, and breast surgeries, although in these cases the risks and benefits must be compared to an epidural. Many different kinds of procedures may benefit from perioperative analgesia provided by PVBs including thoracic surgery, breast surgery, abdominal procedures, and urologic procedures. In addition to use for perioperative analgesia, the PVB has also been used to produce surgical anesthesia. Some centers have had excellent success performing breast procedures under MAC and PVB. Indications:
    - Thoracic surgery
    - Breast surgery
    - Cholecystectomy, upper abdominal surgeries
    - Renal and ureteric surgery
    - Herniorrhaphy, inguinal (T11 to L1 and L2)
    - Appendectomy
    - Colostomy/ileostomy closure
    - Surgical anesthesia
    - Breast surgery, radical mastectomy T1-6, axillary dissection T1-2
    - Herniorrhaphy
    - Chest wound exploration

74. **(C)** Contraindications to PVB include local infection at the site of needle insertion, paravertebral or pleural space infections, and abnormalities of the paravertebral space such as tumors.

A PVB is performed outside the neuraxis, and the risk for spinal hematoma should be minimal with paravertebral block. The use of PVB in patients with mild to moderate anticoagulation has been used in several centers. Because of the potential for needles and catheters to enter the epidural space during an attempted PVB and the potential for bleeding into the paravertebral space, this practice is viewed as controversial by many. To date, there have not been any case reports of severe neurologic injury or bleeding from paravertebral block in anticoagulated patients. Other contraindications include: kyphoscoliosis because the chest deformity may predispose to pleural or thecal puncture; patients with previous thoracotomy that may obliterate the PVS by scar tissue and adhesions of lung to the chest wall; severe hypovolemia, especially for bilateral blocks; and untreated sepsis.

75. (E) A metaanalysis of 10 randomized trials to compare the analgesic efficacy and side effects of paravertebral versus epidural blockade for thoracotomy demonstrated that PVB provided comparable analgesia with epidural blockade after surgery but had a better side effect profile. There was no difference in pain scores between the PVB and epidural groups; however, there was a statistically significant reduction in complications in the PVB group [British Journal of Anaesthesia 2006; 96(4): 418–26]. Single injection produces multidermatomal ipsilateral somatic and sympathetic nerve block, as well as maintains hemodynamic stability, reduces opioid requirements, demonstrates a low incidence of complications (compared to an epidural), preserves bladder sensation, and promotes early mobilization.

76. (A)

77. (F) A PVB injection of local anesthetics results in ipsilateral somatic and sympathetic nerve blocks in multiple contiguous thoracic dermatomes. The spinal nerves in this space are devoid of a fascial sheath, making them susceptible to local anesthetics. If a bolus dose of 20 mL 0.5% bupivacaine is injected, it will result in a maximum concentration of 1.45 mcg/mL in 25 minutes. The accumulation of bupivacaine may occur during continuous paravertebral infusion without clinical signs of toxicity. This accumulation may account for the few reported cases of confusion that resolved after temporary cessation of the infusion. Ropivacaine does not appear to accumulate in the same linear manner as bupivacaine and can be a safer choice for PVB. The absorption of ropivacaine after TPVB is described by rapid and slow absorption phases. The addition of 5 mcg/mL epinephrine to ropivacaine significantly delays its systemic absorption and reduces the peak plasma concentration but its effect on bupivacaine during continuous infusion is unknown. Lidocaine, with a shorter elimination half-life and lower cardiotoxicity than bupivacaine, may be an attractive alternative. Lastly, in cases where pleural integrity is significantly disrupted, alternative means of postthoracotomy analgesia should be considered, as the effectiveness of continuous paravertebral block may be reduced and toxicity may be increased by intrapleural infusion.

78. (E) In the classic landmark based technique, the patient is placed in a sitting position similar to positioning for a thoracic epidural. The spinous processes are marked in the midline, and 2.5 cm lateral to the cephalad edge of the spinous process is marked at the appropriate levels. Infiltration of local anesthesia at the skin entry point is performed prior to advancement of the block needle perpendicular to the skin. The transverse process is usually contacted within 3 to 6 cm. The depth can vary based on the body habitus of the patient and the spinal level. The needle is then walked off the transverse process in a cranial or caudal direction. A cranial direction is preferred because the distance between the superior costotransverse ligament and pleura is longer than when using a caudal angulation; therefore the margin of safety is greater. The skin paravertebral distance is greater at higher and at lower thoracic levels. Body mass index (BMI) significantly influences the distance. In the T7 to T9 region the distance is significantly less influenced by the BMI.

79. Transverse sonogram of the thoracic paravertebral region with the ultrasound beam being insonated between two adjacent transverse processes. Note that the acoustic shadow of the transverse process is now less obvious and parts of the TPVS and the anteromedial reflection of the pleura are now visible. The superior costotransverse ligament (SCL), which forms the posterior border of the TPVS, is also visible and it blends laterally with the internal intercostal membrane, which forms the posterior border of the posterior intercostal space. The communication between the TPVS and the posterior intercostal space is also clearly seen.

80. (A) The lumbar plexus arises for the anterior divisions of the L1 to L4 nerve roots. It may also receive contributions from T12 nerve root in 50% of cases.

81. (B) The lumbar plexus lies most commonly within the posterior one-third of the psoas major muscle, anterior to the transverse processes of the lumbar vertebrae.

82. (A) The lumbar plexus with its six branches covers most of the anterior, medial, and lateral thigh. A lumbar plexus block provides superior analgesia for hip arthroplasty.

83. (B) An intercristal line is drawn at L4/L5 and another line is drawn parallel with the spine through the posterior superior iliac spine (PSIS). The needle is inserted at the intersection of these lines with a slight medial inclination. The needle should be between the transverse processes of L4 and L5 in the landmark Winnie's technique.

84. (D) Semimembranosus and semitendinosus muscles are medial to the nerve. Gastrocnemius muscles are caudad both medially and laterally.

85. (G) Do not confuse local muscle twitches for nerve stimulation. Stimulation of the common peroneal nerve leads to eversion and dorsiflexion of the foot. Stimulation of the posterior tibial nerve is recognized by inversion and plantar flexion of the foot and is the preferred response because it is associated with higher block success; this is an adequate location for the block as long as the stimulation is obtained at least 7 cm cephalad from the popliteal crease. If slight movements of the needle lead to changes in motor response from one nerve to the other, it indicates that you are cephalad to where the sciatic nerve branches. Paresthesias of the medial lower leg occur when stimulating the saphenous nerve.

86. **(B)** The posterior tibial nerve is larger than the common peroneal nerve.

87. **(C)** As the common peroneal and posterior tibial nerves merge, each nerve resembles the weight portion of the dumbbell, and the connective tissue in between the nerves resembles the bar. This sign helps you find the nerves on the ultrasound image. Once the nerves merge and the dumbbell sign disappears, you have reached the sciatic nerve before it divides.

88. **(C)** The popliteal block can be done with the patient in the prone, lateral decubitus, or supine position. Whichever approach you decide to use, the ultrasound image will be the same; it is the needle path and orientation that change. When the patient is prone, lifting your hand upward will direct the needle downward, deeper, and inferior to the sciatic nerve. When the patient is supine, lifting your hand upward will direct the needle downward as well, but this will make it more superficial (closer to the interface of the skin and ultrasound probe) and thus further away from the sciatic nerve. When the patient is supine, you attempt to aim your needle so that it is superior to the sciatic nerve on the ultrasound image.

89. **(B)** For a surgical block of the lower leg, both a popliteal block and an adductor canal block need to be performed. The saphenous nerve is purely sensory and innervates the skin of the medial portion of the lower leg. If a tourniquet were to be placed on the thigh, then for a surgical block, both a subgluteal sciatic and femoral nerve block need to be performed. Ropivacaine 0.2% is a high enough concentration for a sensory block but not a motor block. Ropivacaine 0.5% will provide both a sensory and motor blockade and thus a full surgical block.

90. **(B)** The sciatic nerve is derived from the sacral plexus, and it exits the pelvis from the greater sciatic foramen. It then runs between the greater trochanter and the ischial tuberosity, emerging from deep to the gluteus maximus muscle.

91. **(C)** In a transgluteal sciatic nerve block, the sciatic nerve is visualized in the short axis between the two hyperechoic bony prominences of the ischial tuberosity and the greater trochanter of the femur. The sciatic nerve is located immediately deep to the gluteus muscles, superficial to the quadratus femoris muscle. It is seen as an oval or roughly triangular hyperechoic structure usually found slightly closer to the ischial tuberosity. A high-frequency probe has less depth of penetration but gives better resolution, whereas a low-frequency probe has deeper penetration with low resolution.

92. **(D)** The sciatic nerve is the largest peripheral nerve in the body and is derived from the L4 to S2 nerve roots. In ultrasound-guided high sciatic nerve blocks, the bony landmarks used are the ischial tuberosity and the greater trochanter.

93. (D) The landmarks used in anterior approach to the sciatic nerve block are the anterior superior iliac spine, the pubic tubercle, and the greater trochanter. The posterior cutaneous nerve of the thigh supplies sensory fibers to the posterior part of the thigh and will not be blocked in the anterior sciatic nerve block. The blood vessels lie medial to the nerve and will be injured if the needle is placed too medially.

94. (C) In the anterior approach to sciatic nerve block using ultrasound, a low-frequency probe is used for deeper penetration. It is preferably avoided in patients with coagulopathy as the femoral vessels are at risk of injury. External rotation of the thigh facilitates the block by improving visualization.

95. (B) An ultrasound-guided transgluteal sciatic nerve block is relatively easy to perform with a high success rate. It utilizes the greater trochanter and ischial tuberosity as the bony landmarks. Combined with lumbar plexus block, anesthesia for the entire lower extremity can be achieved. Combined with femoral/saphenous nerve block, anesthesia for the lower limb below the knee can be achieved.

96. (A) In 60 seconds, a 0.1 mL/kg of a local anesthetic solution that contains 5 mcg/cc of epinephrine will result in an increase in the T wave amplitude greater than 25% and ST changes (the most sensitive); and increase in the systolic blood pressure greater than 15 mm Hg; and an increase in the heart rate greater than 10 beats per minute. The remainder of the dose should be injected over several minutes.

97. (B)

Anatomy	Infants	Adults
Spinal cord	L3	L1
Dural sac	S3	S1
CSF/body weight	4 to 6 mL/kg	2 mL/kg

98. (C)

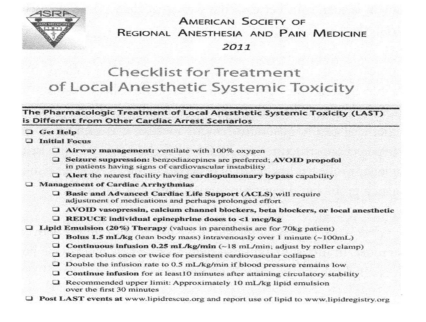

99. (C)   Using a 25# needle directed to each one of the sides of the shaft of the penis (2 and 10 o'clock position), Buck's fascia is pierced. Perform a careful aspiration and use 0.1 mL/kg of bupivacaine 0.25 % at each injection site.

100. (D)   The ilioinguinal and hypogastric nerves originate from the nerve roots of the lumbar plexus (L1) and pass between the transversus abdominis muscle and the internal oblique aponeurosis, near the ASIS. This block is indicated for inguinal herniotomy and orchiopexy procedures and is especially valuable when caudal block is contraindicated or difficult to perform.

101. (D)   The incidence of peripheral nerve injury has remained stable even despite the introduction of ultrasound for a peripheral nerve blockade. The reported frequency of long-term neurologic symptoms after the introduction of ultrasound guidance is virtually identical to that reported from a decade earlier when peripheral nerve stimulation was the primary tool to localize the nerve. In both periods, the reported rate of long-term neurological injury is in the 2 to 4 per 10,000 blocks range. It has been speculated that proximal nerve blocks are riskier than distal approaches. However, there are no convincing data to confirm or refute this notion despite multiple studies. It is, however, believed to be so because proximal nerves contain a higher proportion of neural tissue when compared to connective tissue. Early transient postoperative neurologic symptoms (PONSs) are very common in the first days to month after peripheral nerve blockade. They, however, rarely result in permanent injury. The incidence is reduced with time: 0 to 2.2% at 3 months; 0 to 0.8% at 6 months; and 0 to 0.2% at 1 year. On the other hand, the risk of injury after neuraxial blockade is extremely low, but when they do happen, the injuries are often permanent. Overall, three studies point to an approximate 1 in 8000 incidence of laminectomy after neuraxial blockade, with the risk of permanent injury between 1 in 5800 to 1 in 12,200.

102. (D)   The risk for neuraxial injury, combining hematoma, infection, and direct spinal cord injury, is lower in obstetrical procedures. It is, however, higher in orthopedic surgeries, when there are associated coagulation abnormalities (whether from disease or intended anticoagulation), increased age, and female sex. The risk of hematoma is also higher with epidural than subarachnoid techniques. Concurrent spinal stenosis or some preexisting neurologic diseases may worsen injury severity in the presence of neuraxial hemorrhage or infection. These risk factors are the common themes based on a list of studies reported since 1990.

103. (B)   Epidural and general anesthetics, but not peripheral nerve blocks (PNBs), have been associated with peripheral nerve injury (PNI). PNB is not associated with PNI even after total knee arthroplasty, total hip arthroplasty, or total shoulder arthroplasty. Peripheral nerve injection injury with local anesthetic is greatest when the injection is intrafascicular in location. This is likely related to the exposure of axons to vastly higher concentrations of local anesthetics compared to extraneural application, and mechanical damage to the perineurium and associated loss of the protective environment contained within the perineurium. Tourniquet neuropathy can be associated with marked clinical deficits and pathological changes on electromyography.

104. (D) Shoulder surgeries are most frequently associated with axillary or musculocutaneous nerve injury. The incidence ranges from 0.1% to 10%, most of which are caused by surgical traction to improve exposure or by arthroscopic portal placement. Ulnar neuropathy persists in up to 10% of elbow replacement patients. The common peroneal nerve of the sciatic nerve is most frequently injured during a total hip arthroplasty (0.08% to 3.7%). Injuries to the femoral and superior gluteal nerves are less often. With total knee arthroplasty, the most common injury is to the common peroneal nerve.

105. (C) Local anesthetic, adjuvants, and their combinations have variable effects on spinal cord blood flow (SCBF). The reduction of SCBF in the presence of local anesthetics and adjuvants typically mirrors reduction in metabolic demand secondary to spinal cord anesthesia. There is no evidence that either intravenous or intrathecal epinephrine or phenylephrine adversely affects SCBF. The previously accepted cerebral lower limit of autoregulation (LLA) was 50 mm Hg in humans. Many experts now believe the cerebral LLA in unanesthetized adults is 60 to 65 mm Hg. There is, however, a wide variability of LLA among subjects. Preexisting hypertension seems to be a poor predictor of LLA. The ASRA recommends that blood pressures during neuraxial anesthesia should be maintained in normal ranges or at least 20% to 30% of baseline MAP. When the MAP goes below those parameters, it should not be allowed to persist at those levels. Although these recommended parameters are arbitrary, they are inferred based on large population studies that have linked both degree and duration of hypotension to perioperative cerebral, renal, or myocardial injury. Case reports attest to an extremely small subset of patients who have sustained cerebral or spinal ischemia associated with periods of severe or prolonged blood pressure. Although perioperative occurrence of relative hypotension is common, these rare events stand in stark contrast. It is presumed that the injury does not manifest in most patients because of a physiology reserve that exists between the LLA and blood pressure thresholds below which neurologic injury occurs.

106. (A) Arachnoiditis is a poorly understood diffuse inflammatory reaction of the meninges. Cases of arachnoiditis that stem directly from a neuraxial anesthetic are extremely rare, if they exist at all. There are concerns that antiseptic solutions, particularly chlorhexidine/alcohol mixtures cause arachnoiditis. A retrospective cohort study reported no increased risk in neuraxial complications with the use of chlorhexidine as the skin disinfectant. An in vitro study found chlorhexidine at clinically used concentration is no more cytotoxic than povidone-iodine, and if allowed to dry, any residual chlorhexidine carried by the block needle tip from skin to subarachnoid space would be diluted 145,000 times over. Based on the superiority of chlorhexidine as an antiseptic agent, the ASRA advisory panel stands with other national organizations in recommending it as the skin disinfectant of choice before neuraxial procedures. When used, the chlorhexidine solution should be allowed to completely dry on the skin before needle placement (2 to 3 minutes). The solution should also be physically and temporally separated from block trays and instruments during neuraxial procedures. Care should be taken to avoid needle or catheter contamination from chlorhexidine spraying or dripping or from applicator device disposal onto aseptic work surfaces.

107. (C)   There are no data supporting the use of ultrasound guidance of needle placement reducing the risk of neuraxial injury in patients under general anesthesia or deep sedation. Although warning signs such as paresthesia or pain on injection inconsistently herald needle contact with the spinal cord; nevertheless, some patients do report warning signs of needle-to-neuraxis proximity. General anesthesia or deep sedation abolishes the ability for the patient to recognize and report warning signs. A report from the ASA Close Claims study shows an apparent increase in injury rate in patients who underwent cervical interventional pain medicine procedures under anesthesia or deep sedation. The ASRA advisory panel therefore recommends that neuraxial regional anesthesia should not be performed under general anesthesia or deep sedation in adults. Adults with specific conditions, such as developmental delay or multiple bone trauma, may be appropriate exceptions to this recommendation after considering the risk versus benefit. Conversely, in the pediatric population, the benefit of ensuring a cooperative and immobile infant or child likely outweighs the risk of performing neuraxial regional anesthesia in pediatric patients during general anesthesia or deep sedation.

108. (A)   There are no human data to support the superiority of any nerve localization technique (i.e., peripheral nerve stimulator, injection pressure monitoring, or ultrasound) over another in reducing the likelihood of peripheral nerve injury (PNI). The use of ultrasound enables the detection of intraneural injection. Current ultrasound technology, however, does not have adequate resolution to discern between an interfascicular and intrafascicular injection. Paresthesia during needle advancement or on injection of local anesthetic is not predictive of PNI.

109. (A)   Diabetic polyneuropathy is present in up to 50% of long-standing diabetic patients. Consideration should be given to limiting local anesthetic concentration and/or dose and avoiding adjuvant epinephrine, as these patients may be more sensitive to local anesthetics. Diabetic nerves are less sensitive to electrical stimulation, which theoretically increases risk of intraneural needle placement; thus consideration should be given to ultrasound guidance to maintain needle tip distance from the nerve.

110. (B)   Approximately 30% to 40% of the patients who receive neurotoxic chemotherapeutic agents develop peripheral neuropathy. Many of these neuropathies are subclinical, and the risk of nerve injury is increased further in patients with preexisting neuropathic changes (i.e., diabetes mellitus or alcoholism).

111. (D)   A recent publication reported no evidence that patients with previous spine surgery were at risk for developing new or progressive neurologic deficits when they underwent spinal anesthesia. Neuraxial and interventional pain techniques are not contraindicated in patients with previous spine surgery. Under most clinical circumstances, spinal anesthesia may be both technically easier to perform and more reliable (higher success rates) when compared to epidural anesthesia.

112. (D)   The incidence of iatrogenic direct needle injury or catheter-related injury to the spinal cord is unknown, but is reported to be distinctly rare. Iatrogenic direct mechanical injuries occur by several mechanisms and have been attributed to basic anatomic characteristics of the neuraxis. First, although the termination of the conus medullaris has been commonly described as terminating in the L1 to L2 interspace in adults, its terminus has been found to vary between interspace T12 to L4. Inaccurate identification of a vertebral level during performance of neuraxial anesthesia, especially in patients with obesity, kyphoscoliosis, or previous spinal surgery, further contributes to direct needle and catheter-related spinal cord injury. Second, there may be an incomplete posterior midline fusion of the ligamentum flavum, failing to provide the abrupt change in tissue density clinicians utilize when using the loss-of-resistance technique. Third, because there is a progressive narrowing of the posterior epidural space from caudad (5 to 13 mm in the lumbar region) to cephalad (2 to 4 mm at the low thoracic, 1 to 2 mm at the high thoracic, 0.4 mm at the cervical levels), the margin for error during needle advancement therefore varies at different vertebral levels.

113. (A) Indirect spinal cord injury may result from conditions leading to diminished spinal cord perfusion sufficient enough to cause ischemia. Spinal cord perfusion pressure (SCPP) is determined by the pressure gradient between the mean systemic arterial pressure (MAP) and the cerebrospinal fluid (CSF) pressure [SCPP=MAP−CSF pressure]. SCPP becomes compromised when there is insufficient arterial inflow, inhibited venous outflow, or elevated CSF pressure within the neuraxis. Significant and prolonged systemic hypotension lowers SCPP if CSF pressure is unchanged or elevated. Space-occupying lesions (such as epidural hematoma, abscess, or excessive accumulation of local anesthetics), spinal stenosis, and intradural or extradural masses (such as granulomas that form at the tip of implanted intrathecal catheters) may either exert direct compression on the spinal cord or increase the intrathecal or epidural pressure.

114. (A) Radiologic evaluation of the neuraxis should be considered to better characterize the extent of the tumor. In patients with space-occupying neuraxial lesion near the level of a planned epidural injection, radiologic evaluation of the neuraxis should be considered to better characterize the extent of the mass. Such lesions have been associated with temporary or permanent neurologic deficit due to inadequate neural blood flow, especially when they coexist with epidural space-occupying lesions or processes, such as fluid accumulation within the epidural space. Spinal cord perfusion pressure can be further compromised by prolonged hypoperfusion or certain surgical positions, such as flexed lateral decubitus position.

115. (D) Misidentification of the vertebral level, unrecognized lateral needle placement, challenging surface anatomy, and disease processes that decrease the cross-sectional area within the spinal canal are factors that compromise spinal cord perfusion pressure and have all been associated with adverse neurological outcomes after spinal and epidural anesthetic techniques.

116. (C) Recent studies have found that the lower limit of cerebral and spinal autoregulation in normotensive, unanesthetized adults with intact blood-neural tissue barrier is 60 to

65 mm Hg, higher than the previously accepted MAP range of 50 to 60 mm Hg. There is an existing physiologic reserve that affords some degree of protection during periods of hypoperfusion, which may be significantly compromised by the presence of unrecognized hypertension, increased local tissue pressure, abnormal vascular anatomy, low flow states, disruption of the blood-neural tissue barrier, and impaired carrying capacity of O_2, such as in anemia or erythrocyte sludging.

117. (C) Sickle cell disease may increase the risk of spinal cord ischemia. Preexisting hypertension appears to be a poor predictor of the lower limit of autoregulation, except when systolic pressure is greater than 160 mm Hg. The use of intrathecal or intravenous epinephrine or phenylephrine has not been conclusively shown to have any adverse effects on spinal cord blood flow. Any conditions associated with impaired carrying capacity of O_2 and/ or erythrocyte sludging, such as anemia or sickle cell disease, may increase the risk of injury during and after neuraxial anesthesia. In any instance, when a neuraxial technique is followed by an unexpectedly long period of recovery, unresolved motor weakness, numbness, or block extending beyond the distribution of the intended procedure, reversible causes must be ruled out by reducing or discontinuing local anesthetic infusion, reassessing the patient within an hour, and ordering the appropriate imaging, preferably an MRI, to rule out compressive lesion or spinal cord ischemia. Neurologic consultation is recommended to help evaluate the nature and mechanisms of insults and coordinate further management.

118. (D) In patients on recent bivalirudin therapy, anticoagulant effect should be pharmacologically reversed prior to performance of neuraxial techniques. According to the most recent guidelines for antithrombotic therapy from the American Society of Regional Anesthesia and Pain Medicine (ASRA), dabigatran should be discontinued at least 48 hours before neuraxial injection. Prasugrel should be discontinued at least 7 to 10 days before neuraxial injection. In patients taking fondaparinux, if neuraxial technique has to be performed, single-needle neuraxial technique is recommended, and indwelling catheter placement should be avoided. Recombinant hirudin derivatives are used in cases of heparin-induced thrombocytopenia or as an adjunct when percutaneous angioplasty is performed. The anticoagulant effect of recombinant hirudin derivatives (for example, bivalirudin, lepirudin, desirudin) is present for up to 3 hours after discontinuation of their infusion and cannot be pharmacologically reversed. The most recent ASRA guidelines recommend against neuraxial anesthesia in patients on recent recombinant hirudin derivative therapy.

119. (D) Arachnoiditis is a diffuse inflammatory reaction of the meninges associated most commonly with nonanesthetic conditions, such as trauma, infection, contrast media, or multiple back surgeries. The incidence of arachnoiditis directly stemming from neuraxial techniques is extremely rare. Chlorhexidine has been found superior to povidone-iodine as a disinfectant agent, and its use as an antiseptic of choice before neuraxial techniques is now recommended. According to the ASRA Practice Advisory on Neurologic Injuries, to reduce the risk of chemical arachnoiditis due to skin disinfectants, chlorhexidine/alcohol mixtures should be allowed to fully dry before needle placement, complete physical and temporal separation of disinfectant from the procedural tray should be maintained, and care should be taken to avoid needle or catheter contamination from disinfectant spraying or dripping.

120. (D) Patient characteristics and anesthetic variables are risk modifiers of serious hemorrhagic complications of neuraxial anesthetics. Compared to an atraumatic needle placement in a patient on no preexisting coagulopathy (relative risk: 1.0), the risk of serious bleeding complications is the greatest in instances of traumatic needle placement (RR=112), followed by heparin anticoagulation with concomitant aspirin use (RR=26), traumatic needle placement in patients with no preexisting coagulopathy (RR=11.2). The relative risk of spinal hematoma in patients receiving heparin more than 1 hour after atraumatic needle placement is 2.18 compared to patients not on heparin anticoagulation.

121. (D) When administered intrathecally, clonidine, a centrally acting α_2-receptor agonist, provides analgesic effect by binding to α_2 receptors in the substantia gelatinosa in the spinal cord, binding to the intermediolateral column in the spinal cord, and interacting with excitatory AMPA and inhibitory GABA receptors, with resultant inhibition of substance P release and firing of wide dynamic range neurons in the dorsal horn of the spinal cord. Peripherally it appears to act more like a local anesthetic. With doses between 30 to 300 mcg, clonidine predictably and reliably prolongs the duration of sensory and motor block without having a significant effect on the onset of block. Systemic side effects are hypotension, sedation, and dry mouth. No toxicity was reported with clonidine when administered intrathecally up to 300 mcg.

122. (B) Postdural puncture headache (PDPH) is a common complication of neuraxial anesthesia. The risk of PDPH was found to be lower with epidural anesthesia but may occur in up to 50% in the cases of accidental dural puncture with large-bore epidural needles. PDPH is a characteristically positional, fronto-occipital headache, believed to result from CSF loss through the meningeal needle hole. The incidence of PDPH decreases with increasing age and the use of small-diameter, noncutting spinal needles. Inserting cutting needles perpendicular to dural fibers under longitudinal tension is thought to produce a slit-like dural hole that will pull open under the longitudinal tension of the spinal dura mater. The use of fluid, instead of air, for localizing the epidural space during attempted epidural anesthesia has not been shown to modify the risk of accidental dural puncture, but has been shown to decrease the risk of subsequent PDPH.

Index

Page numbers followed by "*f*" indicate figures.